NOT
YET

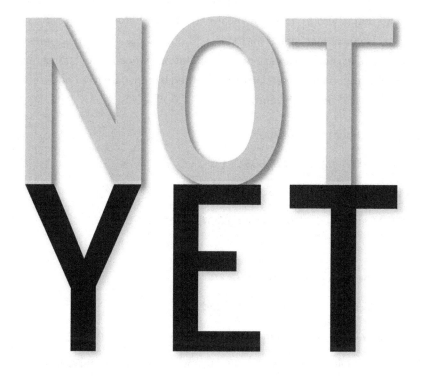

NOT YET

Finding Freedom When Anxiety, Depression, and Other Crap Come Knocking at Your Door

---

TOBY SLOUGH

Published by Cross Timbers Community Church

NOT YET

ISBN (Print Edition): 978-0-9800321-0-9

ISBN (Kindle Edition): 978-0-9800321-3-0

ISBN (Audio Edition): 978-0-9800321-4-7

Library of Congress Control Number (LCCN): 2019918978

Printed in the United States of America

Edited by Wendy K. Walters | www.wendykwalters.com

Published by Cross Timbers Church | www.crosstimberschurch.org

Prepared for publication by Palm Tree Productions | www.palmtreeproductions.com

To contact the author: CTbooks@crosstimberschurch.org

www.tobyslough.com

DEDICATION

FOR GIDDY AND EV
FOR MICAH THOMAS
FOR BUG AND ESSIE

Let me tell you a secret—I wrote *Not Yet* for you. I've been putting off this book for years, and then you five came along. Every time I got to hold each of you for the first time, I looked in your eyes and asked our Father to help you know how much He loves you. A day is coming when life won't go the way that you want it to go and you'll wonder if God is really there, and if He is, does He really care about you. This book is the best gift I could give you for those moments. I hope it's my legacy for you. Your Papa T loves you so very much.

ACKNOWLEDGEMENTS

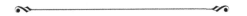

MY CROSS TIMBERS FAMILY—For twenty years you've given Mika and I so much more than we could ever have dreamed. You've given me grace when I don't get it right. You've given me space to be a husband and a dad. You've given me hope in my own battles as I've watched God radically transform your lives. We love you.

JENN DAY—You'll probably try to edit this out when I'm not looking, but you know that I know the truth. This dream would have never come to reality without your passion and tenacity. I am grateful beyond words.

WENDY WALTERS—You are a reminder of a "right on time" God. Your skill is surpassed by only your heart. Mika and I give thanks for you often.

JOHN CHALK—I have no doubt that the strongest relationships are built in the hottest of fires. You are "a brother that's born for adversity" that Solomon was talking about. Thank you, John Boy.

MIKA DI—You are my greatest gift on this planet—nothing else comes close. Watching you love people makes me smile. I love you sweet girl.

PRAISE FOR NOT YET

What happens when what you have been believing for hasn't come? What happens when the thing you know will help you still feels far away? Not afraid of tough topics, Toby opens up the hard conversations many of us are afraid to deal with. *NOT YET* is not a "how to" manual, it is an anthem of faith—even in faith feels far away. I **know** this book will bring people freedom in a way they can't even imagine.

—BIANCA JUAREZ OLTHOFF

Bestselling Author, Pastor, Speaker

NOT YET is one of the most timely and powerful messages I've heard. In a world where anxiety, depression, and fear are rampant—where we often find ourselves desperately searching for our true identity in Christ—this is a "now" book that will help us slow down and re-align our hearts with our Savior. I'm so proud and thankful for Pastor Toby and the vulnerability with which he shares his journey. In this book, he holds nothing back, inviting us to look into some of his darkest days, his deepest depths, and how God redeemed those moments and turned them into hope.

—DINO RIZZO

Author, Speaker, Executive Director of ARC (Association of Related Churches)

Toby Slough is one of my favorite pastors. Not only is he gifted and studied as a teacher, he's as authentic and genuine a person as one could ever hope to know. I feel more loved and seen by Toby and his words than he could ever know. I'm beyond grateful for his work and his life.

—ANNIE F. DOWNS

Bestselling Author, Speaker, Host of That Sounds Fun Podcast

Toby's words won't just bring you help, they will lead you to the hope that there is a God who will rescue you from anything you are going through.

—CARLOS WHITTAKER

Author, Speaker, Moment Maker, Spider Killer, Hope Dealer

If you're tired of wondering why God hasn't moved in your life, wondering if He's forgotten you, done with you, or whether or not he even exists, then *NOT YET* is for you. In these pages, you'll find not only a new, fresh definition of freedom, but through Toby's story, you'll find a path that will illuminate your own path toward healing.

Understanding the concepts of the contents of any book can be insightful and helpful, but knowing the author—the container of the story—is another matter altogether. I've had the privilege of knowing Toby like a second brother for 26 years now. I count it an honor to have had a front-row seat in his cloud of witnesses. To be a part of his healing journey means he's been a part of mine. Toby, thank you for your courage—I pray *NOT YET* will inspire many more to face their Goliaths and find healing in your words.

—BRIAN HACKNEY

Director of Pastoral Care, Cross Timbers Church

I read a great many stories. I like stories. Jesus used stories to convey truth to us, knowing if we could relate to the story, the truth would sink deep and make a difference in our lives. That's what this story does. Toby shares his struggle with such candor that your emotions resonate, chiming in tune with your personal battles, fears, and disappointments. The place to which he has come—knowing God is with him even without his happily ever after—also rings true. It's a relief to know someone else loves God extravagantly and trusts Him completely even without an answer to their deeply held personal desire. You'll find your heart at rest in the comfort and compassion of God at work in your *NOT YET.*

—WENDY K. WALTERS

Author, Ghostwriter, Editor, Speaker

CONTENTS

FROM TOBY'S DAUGHTER

FOREWORD

I remember when dad told me that he worried he wasn't a good enough dad. I didn't understand this at all because, in my eyes, my dad had always been my hero. Growing up, I was always a daddy's girl—even though we did butt heads at times! We both are passionate people, and I always thought I was right, so you can imagine how that usually turned out. But it's funny how your perspective on your childhood changes as you get older and have kids of your own. I realize that I didn't make it easy for my parents. When I look back, I remember my dad always showing me so much grace and love despite the things I said or did. I remember him apologizing when he might have said something he didn't mean. I know he is not perfect, but he has always been the epitome of love and acceptance.

The story in this book explains why.

The person I knew at home was always the same person who stood on that stage at church. He was never trying to act like he had it all together or be someone that he's not after the church doors close and everyone goes home. He's always been real and vulnerable and shared his struggles openly but he never really brought me into his world of panic and anxiety. I didn't know some of the stories in the pages to follow until I was in college and heard him open up during a sermon. He sheltered my brother and me from that, and I understand why. He didn't want us to have the same struggles he had. It wasn't until I started battling my worries and fears that I began to understand what he had gone through and how the Lord was still redeeming the dark moments.

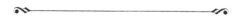

I can still visualize that day, sitting in the recliner in our apartment in Mississippi. My husband, Grant, and I had only lived there for a few months. Grant worked super long hours, so I was often home alone in this new place. I was in between jobs, and I had very few real friends. I don't even know what started it all that day, but my mind just felt out of control, spiraling downward, and I couldn't seem to snap out of it. I felt like I didn't have a purpose, like I was not a good wife, like I was about to go crazy, and that no one understood. Looking back, it seems silly, but it felt very real to me. My dad was the first person I called.

He wasn't a stranger to struggle and battles within the mind, so I always felt safe with him. I couldn't explain how I felt. I didn't know how to put it into words but he sat and listened as I cried. He didn't try to figure it out. He told me I was not crazy and reminded me of who God says I am. Then he suggested I talk to a counselor. At first, I felt embarrassed. I told him that seeing a counselor made me feel like I had failed, like I hadn't relied on Jesus enough. Dad said, "Bailey, It doesn't mean you've failed at all. His Spirit can work through people, and you don't have to go through this alone. I know,

I've been there. I'll call you right back." Not even fifteen minutes later, my phone rang, and dad told me he had called a friend in Louisiana who knew a trusted Christian counselor not too far from me and that I had an appointment scheduled later that day. And that's when the Lord began to take me down my path towards freedom and healing.

As a father, he would have never chosen for me to understand some of what he goes through personally. I know that because he has told me. And as a daughter, I still pray God will take away this ongoing battle in his mind. But I've watched time and time again the way his story and the fact he is living in the "not yet" has impacted so many lives.

I am reminded of what Paul said:

> Therefore, my dear brothers and sisters, stand firm. Let nothing move you. Always give yourselves fully to the work of the Lord, because you know that your labor in the Lord is not in vain.[1]

I know for a fact that my dad is giving himself entirely to the work of the Lord, and sharing this story is one huge piece of it. His pain is not in vain, and neither is yours.

—*Bailey Slough Garner*

ENDNOTE

1. 1 Corinthians 15:58.

INTRODUCTION

YOU HAVE TO PLAY SCARED

My future was in the National Football League—of this one thing I was certain. I was twelve years old, eighty pounds soaking wet (maybe), and one of the three fastest guys in my class at Northside Elementary. We had begun our first year of junior high football in shorts and t-shirts, running wind sprints, doing agility drills, and getting to know the guys coming up from the two other elementary schools in town. After a week of general conditioning and orientation, it was finally time to put on the pads. I could hardly sleep the night before—I had dreamed of this day since my mom had pulled my brother and me in the wagon to watch Dad coaching on Friday nights. I fell asleep with dreams of autograph signings and cheering fans in the days ahead.

Morning came. We suited up, jogged out on the field, and after a few warmups exercises we lined up for our first tackling drill. I got in the running back line, took the handoff, and gave an unbelievably athletic juke to a kid from Eastside Elementary that I had just met the day before. I had a derogatory comment for the kid and a big grin for the coach as I jogged over to the tackling line. "Slough, you're up next!" the coach said, and there stood Kenneth with the ball in his arms, just looking down at me, just shaking his head.

Kenneth Johnson. Westside Elementary. No matter which school you had attended, everyone knew Kenneth. Almost six feet tall, the chiseled body that looked like one of those Greek god statues we had seen in history class, *and* a goatee—Kenneth Johnson was a legend. There was an audible "Oooh" from the guys in line, and I noticed the dads moving in closer to watch what happened. It's a moment frozen in time that I remember like it was yesterday. A moment of panic set in as the thought crossed my mind, *I might get seriously hurt here.* The only thing scarier than the paramedics showing up was the distinct possibility that I might get laughed off the field in front of my teammates, the coaches, and that word would get back to Dad.

The whistle blew. Kenneth moved forward, and I had one of those out of body experiences where my brain said advance and my legs wouldn't cooperate. I actually started to retreat. The guys laughed, the coach blew his whistle and the coach yelled, "Do it again!"

Same whistle. Same result.

Kenneth yelled out, "What's wrong with you? You scared? Hit me!"

We lined up a third time and ... yep, I backed up once again. I walked to the back of the line with my eyes on the ground, the laughter of my teammates ringing in my ears. The dreams of autographing signings and television interviews died on a sticker-filled football field in Angleton, Texas.

I learned a great lesson that day. If you don't learn how to move forward when your knees are shaking and the possibility of failure seem likely, your worst nightmare might become your reality. Life is about learning how to play scared. Little did I know how much that truth might become my reality later in life when the stakes were much higher than a football game. My life and the life of my family would hang in the balance.

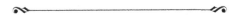

The story of the prodigal son in Luke 15 is one of the most familiar stories in all the Bible. At its core, it's a story of rebellion and grace— the selfishness of a son and the unconditional, radical love of a father. But it's also a story of courage. I'm sure you've heard it: an ungrateful boy takes his part of his family's inheritance and wastes it on fast women and fast chariots. The cash runs out, his "friends" run off, and the boy born with a silver spoon in his mouth finds himself wrestling pigs for the scraps in the bottom of the bucket just to get by. Desperate, ashamed and out of options, he decides to throw a Hail Mary pass. His plan is to go home and ask his dad for a job alongside the very men who had served him his entire life.

He makes the shame-filled journey home and finds his father pacing the porch. The moment he sees his son, dad runs to meet him, gives him his credit card, and throws a party to welcome him home. Like every great story, the ending is the best part. But pause in the middle with me. Put yourself in the pig urine-soaked sandals of the boy who finds himself in the mess of his own making. Did he think the plan would work? Do you honestly think that on his way home, the boy was saying to himself, "Man, they're going to write a book about this someday?" His future was uncertain at best. That walk defines playing scared.

The courage born out of desperation when you find yourself living in the "not yet" moments of life is powerful and possible. Because if you take a step when your pain tells you that you don't have one left in you, there's a loving Father at the end of the journey waiting to embrace you with a ring and a robe and welcome you back into the family. Sometimes you have to play scared.

THE COURAGE BORN OUT OF DESPERATION WHEN YOU FIND YOURSELF LIVING IN THE "NOT YET" MOMENTS OF LIFE IS POWERFUL AND POSSIBLE

I know your time is valuable, so let me try to save you some. If you're a formula kind of person who is looking for some "3 Easy Steps to a Better Life Plan" to solve your challenges, you might want to close this one and keep looking. If your picture of a pastor is one of a near-perfect performer who has the answers to all of your questions, I'm not your man. It's probably not for you. Who's it for? Glad you asked.

Not Yet is for all of you who fight feelings of being "less than." You're living in a pigpen, and whether it's from your poor decision making or someone else's, you're desperate for someone to throw you a lifeline. It's for the divorced dad who never gets to see his kids. It's for the single mom who lays down at night wondering where she'll get the strength to make it another day. It's for the business leader who, by all appearances, has it all but lays in bed at night wondering why his world is spinning out of control. It's for the college girl who knows she shouldn't measure her worth by comparing herself to the airbrushed images of Instagram but doesn't have a clue how to stop that train from leaving the station. It's for every person whose image of Jesus has been tainted by a Christian teacher, leader, or friend who made them feel like the problem was a lack of faith. It's for the guy or girl who hasn't had their biggest prayers answered and have convinced themselves, "Either something is wrong with me or something is wrong with God because this Jesus thing just doesn't seem to work for me." And it's for the thousands of people just like me who love Jesus and suffer from panic attacks, anxiety, or depression and find themselves wondering what in the hell God is up to.

Not Yet is about not beating yourself up for being scared but learning how to live with courage and freedom when life calls you to play scared. It's about discovering the truth about God and how He is at work in the most unlikely "un-churchy" kind of things. It's about discovering a Father who is not standing far off somewhere waiting for you but walking with you, right in the middle of your brokenness and mess.

This is my story. Let's begin when it all fell apart.

CHAPTER ONE

A BRIDGE OVER 1-35

Daydreams are weird. You can't plan them. They happen when they happen and without much rhyme or reason. There you are, conscious and alert, when seemingly out of nowhere—your mind goes somewhere else. Most of the time, you don't even know you're daydreaming until you wake up and catch yourself in that thought. My usual reaction at that moment is, "Wow, why did I think about that?" I don't remember many of my daydreams; they just come and go. But for one particular daydream, that was not the case.

It was a hot June afternoon in Texas—95° in the shade with 150% humidity in the air. My car's air conditioner was running at maximum of maximum, and the temperature inside wasn't far from the temperature of a refrigerator. Although it was almost cold enough to hang meat, it wasn't cooling me off at all. Sweat was dripping off my mostly bald head, mingling with the tears and snot running down my face. I was gripping the steering wheel with Tom Cruise-hanging-off-a-building strength. *Mercy Came Running* was blaring through the speakers at an ear-rattling volume for the tenth time in a row. My heart was beating fast (again). I was doing 70 mph in a 55-mph zone headed south on Interstate 35 when I started daydreaming. I'm not sure how long it lasted, but I "woke up" and caught myself in this thought: *If I hit that bridge abutment doing 70 mph, would Mika know that I did it on purpose?*

This time, I didn't have to wonder why I was thinking that thought. I knew exactly why I was daydreaming about leaving this life behind.

I had reached my breaking point.

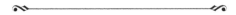

It was 1996, and I was finally living the dream of pastoring church, a desire of mine since my senior year in college. My wife, Mika, and I lived in the perfect place for a couple of Texas-born and raised kids: the Dallas/Fort Worth area. I had a crazy sweet and gorgeous wife, a nine-year-old, beautiful, blonde-headed daughter named Bailey, and a seven-year-old, full-of-life son, Ross. For almost four years, I had been teaching the Bible and serving our church family. God was blessing us with growth. We had doubled in size, and enthusiasm was high. Life was really good, and my future was filled with unlimited opportunities. At least, that is how it seemed to everyone around me. What no one knew was that I hadn't slept for more than thirty minutes segments at a time for the past seventeen days.

Late that evening, we turned in for the night. Mika is blessed with the "those-who-trust-in-you-will-rest-in-perfect-peace" kind of sleep. Before her head is fully compressed in the pillow, she's in full REM. That night my bridge moment was weighing heavily on my mind, and as I listened to Mika's rhythmic breathing, my heart began to pound. As my heartbeat raced up, my breath came faster and then faster. My first thought was, *I'm having a heart attack.* Fear gripped me, but at that moment, it wasn't a heart attack I was afraid of. My terror was because I didn't have a clue about what was happening to me. I felt like I was out of control.

After about ten minutes of intense panic, I decided to get up and walk the little hallway of our house and try to wear myself out. (I'm not a physician, but I play one on TV!) From 11:00 that night until 4:30 the next morning, I walked that hallway—crying, bargaining with God, begging Him, reciting every Bible verse I knew—I just kept walking. Finally, exhausted, defeated, terrified, and sweating like a guy who had just finished an ultra-marathon, I laid down beside my wife, closed my eyes, and dozed off. I slept for about thirty minutes. This night was the first of seventeen. For seventeen straight days, I didn't sleep, I barely ate, and walked what must have equaled miles up and down our hallway. I was significantly sleep deprived. I was experiencing stress like I had never known. I lost almost twenty pounds. Walking most of the night and throwing up most of what you eat will do that to you.

Those days were excruciating. I had a special drill I ran through to get me through my workday. On Sundays, I would get in my car to drive to the church. On the way, I would pull over on the side of the road and throw up. Once I made it to church, I would lay my head down on my desk and sob. I would tell God that there was no way I could get up in front of a room full of people and preach. Then someone would knock on the door, and it would be time to go. Somehow, I always managed to walk out, stand behind the pulpit, and preach. I don't know how I did it. It was a different kind of teaching, not delivered out of joyful revelation, but out of utter desperation. When I finished with one service, I would go back to my office, lay my head on my desk, and begin to cry again. Mika would come in between the services to pray over me and give me a verse. Then I would go out and do it all over again. This sad song was on repeat for months. I wondered, *God, how in the world could you call me to ministry and yet allow me to face this battle?*

I tried making deals with God. I told Him, "Lord, if you will pull me out of this … if you will just let me sleep again, eat again, start to function again … I promise, I'll tell the truth about the battle I faced, and I'll do my best to help others who are fighting the same battle." I would like to say that God delivered me overnight but that wasn't the case. What I can tell you is that He did start me down an incredible road to freedom.

No one will ever convince me that God isn't in the miracle business. I experienced two during those seventeen days. The first was that I didn't run into the I-35 bridge support that day. It took everything I had to stay in my lane, but I've since come to know it wasn't really me at all. It was His power working through His grace that kept me from doing the unthinkable. The longer I live, the more I realize I don't have enough power to do anything. It is His power. Even when I was convinced that I had run out of options, and the father of lies was whispering some outrageous crap in my ear that sounds ridiculous today but seemed very real in my moment of pain, God was at work in me. Only the Truth-Giver could give me what I needed that day.

The second miracle was that I was able to keep that seventeen days a secret from my wife and those close to me. As painful as it is to type—hiding the truth was my ultimate goal—and I was good at pretending. I was really good at it. Good enough to hide the hell I was living in from the very ones who loved me the most; they were also the ones best positioned to help me find freedom. Satan is a master at deception, convincing me that hiding was protection. But the isolation I subjected myself to was wreaking havoc on my emotional well-being. Those seventeen days were a dark season I don't want to relive, but as I reflect, I can see God's presence in the darkness of those days. Do you need to hear that today? Do you need to hear that even in your darkness, He is with you?

Nearly two weeks passed before I sat in a counselor's office for the first time. It was in that first visit that I heard the words *panic attack* and *anxiety disorder*. Here I was, a type-A, hard-driving, mountain-taking kind of guy, and I had to stop. Those seventeen days forced me to stop and look inside myself. The journey had begun, and like most journeys, it would be a zigzag of a ride—back and forth, ups and downs, highs and lows. Through the process, I've learned some things, unlearned some things, and finally come to peace with the fact that I will never arrive. The destination is the not point; it's what He shapes me into on the journey that matters.

I've hesitated, put off, and rationalized away writing this book for years. I've had lots of excellent reasons—many of which you'll read about in the pages ahead. The biggest thing that has held me back for so long is my search for a way to articulate my story in a way that helps those of you who struggle with something that isn't panic or anxiety. Although my battle with panic and anxiety is real and my only personal illustration for what I'm trying to share, it's not the whole war. The war is bigger than that. The war is about the lie I began to believe in the middle of the battle: the lie that *I am not enough*.

Not *good* enough.

Not *holy* enough.

Not *strong* enough.

Not *faith-filled* enough.

My condition became so severe that I firmly believed everything I held dear was going to be taken away. I was afraid I would lose my wife, my kids, and my ministry. Looking back, I see that those thoughts were unwarranted and irrational, but at the time they seemed like concrete realities. You see, that's the root of the root. Your issue, condition, limp, whatever you want to call it, can isolate you. Satan whisper lies in your ear, rips at your heart, weakens your faith, and causes you to stumble. There was no reason for me to believe bad things would happen, yet I was convinced they would. Fear controlled my mind which caused my emotions to react violently. The brain cannot distinguish the difference between a real physical threat and an emotional or perceived one. Our bodies respond to anxiety with the same wash of fight, flight, or freeze chemicals they release if you were being attacked by a lion or bear. Fear is nothing but a liar, and it sells a lie your body buys. Prolonged anxiety shreds the body, and mine was being destroyed.

> THERE WAS NO REASON FOR ME TO BELIEVE BAD THINGS WOULD HAPPEN, YET I WAS CONVINCED THEY WOULD

As I look back on those dark days, I know God was with me. I see how He provided for me through my wife, Mika. God has empowered her to minister to me in remarkable ways. Some of the sweetest moments of my life are the times when she would pray over me, pray for me, and read scripture at three o'clock in the morning when I was sobbing uncontrollably.

Ironically, though, while Mika was a great source of comfort, she was also one of my most significant sources of stress. Yes, she was always there for me. Yet even with all her compassion and love, it was hard for her to grasp what I was experiencing. I would use all the analogies I could think of to try to help her understand, but she couldn't possibly understand it all. It was hard for me to articulate, so she would try and say things that would help. She would give me ideas on what she thought I could do to help but the things she said tended to make things worse. I hated that for us. As much as she loved me and as much as I needed her to understand, we couldn't bridge the disconnect. We had almost always been on the same page, but this battle was different than anything we had experienced. It was incredibly painful knowing that the one I loved the most had no frame of reference by which to grasp the enormity of my struggle. This reality made what I was experiencing even more difficult.

One of the key pieces of my anxiety puzzle was revealed when I began to realize was that I wanted some assurance in life. I desperately needed 100% guarantees that things would work out the way I wanted them to work out. My tremendous need to control all the things in my life was causing high levels of anxiety. As I worked my way through this sobering truth, one of the verses the Lord gave was:

> *Everything in the heavens and on earth is Yours, O Lord, and this is your kingdom. We adore you as the one who is over all things.*[1]

While God had given Mika to me to be a wonderfully loving and supportive wife, He was still to be my satisfaction. My rest, my comfort, and my peace were to come from Jesus, not Mika. Grasping this was a real turning point for me, and a major part of the healing process was beginning to understand how I depended on her for things she was not designed to give me.

It was a long road, but over time, God brought liberation from the binding chains of anxiety. It was torturesome, but in that pain, I learned an essential truth:

> That is why we never give up ... For our present troubles
> are quite small and won't last very long. Yet they produce
> for us an immeasurable great glory that will last forever!"[2]

This truth takes me back to the prodigal son. By the time he realized he was in trouble, he was out of money and resources. The friends he had partied with were long gone, and he didn't know where to go to get help. So, to survive, he got a job feeding pigs. This didn't solve all his problems, though; he was still hungry. His next attempt at trying to fix things was begging to eat some of the pig's slop, but they turned him down. No matter what he tried, he could not seem to find an answer to his problems. Many times, we are taught that the lesson we can learn from the prodigal son is to not be greedy, to not be spoiled. I think the prodigal son wanted control. He wanted what he thought was best for him how he wanted it and when he wanted it. In a way, he wanted to be his own god—his own little "g" god. Once he took matters into his own hands, he felt the world turn its back on him. He felt alone. Like me, he felt like he was out of options. He was completely out of control.

Your issues can lead you to some very dark places. It feels like God has turned His back on you, like He has written you off as a lost cause. Nobody seems to grasp what you are going through. The tunnel is long and dark, and there is no light at the end of it. But those are all lies.

Let me give you some good news: God hears your desperate cries and has already made a way for your deliverance. The answer to your question has already been given. The work it took to free you from this prison has already been done. Jesus came to set you free! God never intended His children to live in bondage, fear, or worry. He wants your heart to be glad and your life to be full. His dream for you is so much greater than you can ever imagine.

The solution does not lie in a pill, a chant, or any other quick-fix remedy. It won't come by your hard work, by pulling yourself together, gritting your teeth, or whatever you think you can do on your own to make it go away. You can set your mind to get rid of your "thing" but in your own strength it is impossible. Most likely, your path to freedom will not be an easy one. But be sure, be certain, that Jesus knows the way because He paved the way. It is your job to follow Him and learn to walk the path. At times, this path may seem long and complicated, but as one who has been where you are and is now living in freedom, let me encourage you with this: you can be thankful for every step of the journey. Each step has purpose. There is promise in your pain. I thank Him for my journey. The work He did on my behalf has blessed me through the fight and far beyond the struggle. Know that there is hope for your troubled heart.

Anxiety is primarily an issue of control. So, my question to you is this: "Who is in control?" If you have been on track with me so far, the odds are good that fear controls you. Fear gains control over your mind by convincing you that you know the best way to manage everything in your life. Once you buy into this lie, you realize then that there is no way you can make your "perfect" plan happen, and the "what if" game begins. Soon you become exhausted by worrying about the uncontrollable answers.

> ANXIETY IS PRIMARILY AN ISSUE OF CONTROL

- ***What if*** things don't go as I planned?

- ***What if*** I don't get the promotion I know I deserve?

- ***What if*** my daughter doesn't choose the college I know is best for her?

- ***What if ...?***

Jesus asks this:

> "Are you tired? Worn out? Burned out on religion? Come to me. Get away with me and you'll recover your life. I'll show you how to take a real rest. Walk with me and work with me—watch how I do it. **Learn the unforced rhythms of grace.** I won't lay anything heavy or ill-fitting on you. **Keep company with me and you'll learn to live freely and lightly.**"[3]

I know what it feels like to not sleep for seven ... eight ... twelve ... seventeen days. I know what it feels like to be covered in shame and worthlessness because my life was out of control. My story is filled with disappointments, detours, unanswered prayers ... and lots of questions. It's also filled with the undying belief that God shows up in the *Not Yet* moments and does what only He can do.

Your struggle may not be an emotional issue. Yours may be relational or physical. Your divorce, addiction, bankruptcy, or disease may have left you vulnerable to the lie that you are not enough—that if you were better, or if God was real, this would all be fixed.

I invite you to commit to keep reading. Commit to take another step. This book may not be easy for you to read. It may be difficult for you to believe in the hope I am telling you about. I have come a long way since that day on 1-35. God has been faithful with every step I took, and I am believing for you when you can't believe for yourself. My prayer is that you will find a new definition of freedom.

Here we go.

ENDNOTES

1.   1 Chronicles 29:11.
2.   2 Chronicles 4:16-17.
3.   Matthew 11:29-30, MSG, (author emphasis).

GOD SHOWS UP IN
OUR *NOT YET* MOMENTS
AND DOES WHAT
ONLY HE CAN DO

CHAPTER TWO

THE PRISON SENTENCE

The life of twelve-year-old boys in my South Texas town was one big game of "King of the Hill." It had been that way for generations. Anyone on the top of the hill had to fight to keep from having to share their place. Of course, there were fights to stay on top of the hill, but our version was not exactly like the way others played the game. Being the "king" was not just about brute strength and might. For my group, sports determined who stood proudly at the top. Baseball was king at that point in our lives. The ability to hit, run, catch, and throw a baseball determined your place in the pecking order. Performing was everything. Selection to the annual All-Star team stamped you with a gold star of approval among the guys. The problem for me was not the team. Being around a bunch of guys was the ideal way to spend springs and summers. My conflict came because All-Star games were Wednesday night affairs, and we went to church on Wednesday nights—*no* exceptions. I was a very competitive kid, plus I had an older brother. Making the team wasn't an issue, however, convincing my dad to let me miss church on Wednesday nights to play baseball was an insurmountable problem.

"I'm sorry, son, but you are already committed on Wednesdays," my father told me. My heart sank. The high of making the team was squelched by my father's pre-established Wednesday night appointments. That night I *should* have been in bed dreaming of fly ball snags and grand slam home runs. Instead, my eyes were filled with real tears rolling down my face. Yes, I wanted to play on that All-Star Team, and I wanted to be around my buddies that wanted to do the same thing. However, my heart stopped just short of celebration. The fact that I wanted to play baseball rather than go to the church filled me with a sense of shame that, at the time, I couldn't possibly understand.

Good boys would never choose baseball over God was the lie I fell asleep believing that night. *I must not be a good boy then*, and just like that, a genuine acceptance of a lie over something as insignificant as baseball began an erroneous belief system that would stay with me most of my adult life. It was the beginning of me truly wondering if I would ever be good enough for God. More than thirty years would pass before I was ready for God to show me how much that lie had not only marked me but how much the lie wreaked havoc in my life.

Baseball wasn't the only place where performance was a priority. Church was another form of the "King of the Hill" game. Sunday school lessons led me to believe that boys with the best behavior made God happy. Bad boys made Jesus and Sunday school teachers very sad, and I will be the first to admit that I made Jesus sad—a LOT! I don't even want to venture to guess how I made my Sunday School teachers feel. Most of the time, I considered myself to be a bad boy trying really hard to be a good boy. The thing I felt most successful at was falling short all the time. To be good felt like being in a pickle between third base and home plate. I became a champion at putting pressure on myself.

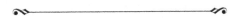

One Sunday, when I was in my early teens, we were attending service just like most every Sunday morning. This particular Sunday, I vividly remember watching one of the leaders of our church stand up and announce the sins of another member of our church. I don't remember the exact words or party language, but I was sure that from this day in time, this accused man was to be considered a very bad boy. We were instructed to "have nothing to do with him." This once beloved son was now denounced. Blackballed. He would most likely never find his way back to the top of any of our hills. Later, the Sunday lunch conversations among my uncles, aunts, and cousins were centered around the scarlet letter announcement. The proper response was decided. If by any chance we were to run into THAT man in our little town, we would not give him the time of day.

We were told not to speak to him. We were to refrain from any and all interaction with him. He was not a part of our sacred circle anymore. That afternoon and late into the evening, I was literally tormented with the aftershocks of the announcement. My mind tried to comprehend this candid and open discussion surrounding this respected man's fall from grace. My heart struggled to navigate the abrupt and sudden end to his place as a king in our community. I asked myself the question, *If it could happen to someone like him, what would I have to do to keep it from happening to me?* My stomach sank with the realization, *Whatever "it" was, I was probably not "whatever" enough.*

That night, I laid in bed and wondered when the day would come when there would be other families sitting around their Sunday lunch table talking about me. In my heart, it seemed inevitable. I knew there was no safeguard to keep me from messing up. I was sure that a fall from the hill was right around the corner for me. I was keenly aware of the dark places in my soul as well as the mistakes that I was making day after day. *Would people be judging the worst decisions of my life?* I made a mental list of all the mistakes that I made. I sidelined all the excuses I could have given myself. I examined each scenario with a magnifying glass, systematically studying the details of my wayward ways. I was that baseball boy all over again. I felt like the choices I had made would keep God from being happy with me.

I was acutely aware of my errors and simultaneously filled with shame. Somewhere during that season of my life, I began to believe that if I were ever fully known, I would never be fully loved. One by one, I started to set in place the bars of my own self-imposed prison. Lie by lie, I built a jail cell on the dangerously sandy foundation that performance equals acceptance. I was becoming more miserable by the day. The ironic thing was, it felt spiritual to me. Beating myself down began to feel holy. The more miserable I felt about myself, the more worthy I believed I was becoming. The unhealthy disciplines required to be a "good boy" were being etched like stone in my ever-hardening heart. I had drawn foul ball lines in every direction, and I was determined to live in between them. I knew that if I prayed hard enough, if I hung out with just the right people, if I did this, if I didn't do that ... surely, I could become good enough.

> I BEGAN TO BELIEVE THAT IF I WERE EVER FULLY KNOWN, I WOULD NEVER BE FULLY LOVED

Performance.

Good enough.

Control.

Better.

My prayer became, "God, please help me do better."

My internal response to my prison sentence was to put my head down and try harder. The desire to achieve, to be the one at the top of the hill, was in my DNA. The way to be accepted was to **do better**. I was an extroverted, driven kid who believed, "If you're not first, you're last." My mother and father would have really *loved* it if I had felt that way about my schoolwork (which was not the case)! On the inside I felt like a failure every single day, but I was always able to hide my insecurities behind my outgoing personality. I was in for anything that made me liked and accepted by my teammates and friends.

I was part of a high-achieving family. My mother was an elementary school teacher, and my father was a high school coach. We had expectations in our family, just like the majority of other families. Some were spoken, and some were just understood. My father raised my brother and I like practically every coach led their teams in the '60s and '70s. I call it the "you can do better" approach.

"Son, that was a great forty split, but *I think you can do better*."

"Son, that was a great tackle, but *I think you can do better*."

"Son, that was a great catch out there, but *I think you can do better*."

"I think you can, but if you can't, I can find someone who can."

The truth was, a lot of the time, and in many situations, I could have done better. I could have practiced a little longer in the evenings. I could have studied a little harder at night. I could have applied myself a bit more during the school day. I could have asked for tutoring or help when my grades started to slip. But I didn't do any of those good things that could have helped me. My dad is an amazing man, and there is no doubt that he loved me and wanted the best for me. I don't really recall asking my mom for help with grades either. Internally, I told myself that it was up to me to get it right. I believed that asking mom or dad for anything would clue them in to the fact that I was really a failure. They would know my secret, and I was too ashamed of who I was to let them know the truth about how I was struggling.

Looking back, I know I was a challenge to raise. I wasn't anywhere near perfect, and I knew it. But if you combine a deeply held insecurity covered up by an outgoing personality with a "more, better, faster" kind of parenting style, you get a kid who starts believing that he will *never* be good enough. I knew my dad loved me, but somewhere deep down inside, I was convinced that I was a source of disappointment to him. This was the theme of my years in high school. I will never forget the day I left for college; Dad stood there with tears running down his cheeks. I drove away thinking to myself, *I am going to show my dad that I can be something. He's going to be proud of me one day.* College was my next big chance to **do better**.

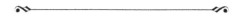

Is there where you find yourself? Do you feel like you have something to prove? You're not alone. I've met many men and women who have been through the rejection of a divorce and are spending their days trying to prove to their former spouse and to others that they are worthy. I've met others whose mom or dad left when they were little, and somewhere down in their heart, they decided that it was their fault. One of my dear friends told me she began drinking when she was eleven to numb the pain of having a mother that didn't love or value her. So many from my generation have made poor life decisions in a desperate attempt to hear an authority figure in their lives say, "Way to go!" One of the big problems with this way of thinking is that we never reach our destination. There is always another mountain to climb. It's never good enough when you are hearing the voice of a dad or a mate or a friend saying, "Is that best you can do?"

Culture isn't helping: our world applauds and esteems a driven lifestyle and the achievement that comes with it. Many times, in my opinion, the church exacerbates the issue. The culture of "shooting our own wounded" is a persistent problem. This isn't a new problem in the church community. It's just one that needs to come to an end. Gossip in "prayer circles" and dinner tables lead hurting people to live with the fear of being the subject of the next gathering. We're still shaming others. It may not be as overt as a "have nothing to do with this man" statement, but any issue with mental or emotional health is seen by too many as a lack of faith. The subtle message of "perform or be rejected" continues to be alive and well. There's too much "you need to" and not enough "me too" simmering in our sermons and blog posts.

My experience tells me that if you're operating out of a mindset that says, "not good enough," every success brings more pressure to do more, to be more; because if they ever figure out who you really are, the whole house of cards comes toppling down.

Acceptance was my ultimate goal, and an idol for me became the happiness of others. It began with my dad, then it projected onto other father figures in my life and evolved into the insane effort to make sure everyone was happy with me. Making others happy isn't a bad thing but living your life for the acceptance of others is called the fear of man in the Bible, and it's a trap. I know this trap well.

I've been blessed to be a part of two growing ministries in my adult life. Growth is good, but if performance is your goal, growing churches just mean more opinions to weigh and more people to please. I found myself lying in bed "replaying the tapes" in my head of conversations that I should have handled differently, sermons that I should have preached better, ways that I was failing as a husband and a father. The more public our ministry became, the more pressure I felt. At some level, I was afraid to enjoy my life. I didn't feel as if I deserved any joy and being spiritual meant being miserable. I was trapped, and I didn't know how to get out.

THE MORE PUBLIC OUR MINISTRY BECAME, THE MORE PRESSURE I FELT

My "thorn in the flesh" is an anxiety/panic disorder and the battle with depression that inevitably comes on the heels of those attacks. Your thorn may be an emotional health issue like mine, or it may be something from an entirely different category. Some of you may have health challenges or money problems or are living through the hell of a divorce. You may have a son or daughter that you haven't talked to in years or a battle with lust or an addiction you can't seem to find victory over. No matter what category you place your "thorn" in, the result is the same: you feel "less than." You feel *less than* the co-worker, the neighbor, the friend, or the couple that sits in the seats in front of you at church every (or almost every) Sunday.

It took me years to realize that my problem is not my problem. Stay with me here. I'm not saying that the challenges I've listed above (and many others) aren't real challenges. I'm not implying that God doesn't want to bring healing into your situation. What I AM saying is that my real problem is not an anxiety issue, it's the lies I am prone to believe when the pain of that thorn comes crashing into my life. Lies like:

- I'm "less than," if I just read my Bible more, prayed more, loved God more, I wouldn't fight this battle.

- My panic attacks are an indicator of my level of faith, and if people knew the depths of my depression, the irrational nature of my thoughts in the middle of a panic attack, they'd have nothing to do with me.

- I'm a burden to my wife, my kids, my staff and leaders, and our church.

Pain produces fear, and fear is a liar! Paul said that his thorn was given to him to humble him—humility is a beautiful thing. But the thorn God brought or allowed (Does it matter? It's a thorn, and it hurts!) mixed in with lies from the pit of hell can destroy you if you believe those lies long enough.

This anxiety/panic battle depleted me emotionally, physically, and spiritually. Let's return to Jesus talking about a son who ran out of options:

> There was a man who had two sons. The younger one said
> to his Father, "Father, give me my share of the estate." So, he
> divided his property between them.

Not long after that, the younger son got together all he had, set off for a distant country and there squandered his wealth in wild living. After he had spent everything, there was a severe famine in that whole country, and he began to be in need. So, he went and hired himself out to a citizen of that country, who sent him to his fields to feed pigs. He longed to fill his stomach with the pods that the pigs were eating, but no one gave him anything.

When he came to his senses, he said, "How many of my father's hired servants have food to spare, and here I am starving to death! I will set out and go back to my father and say to him: Father, I have sinned against heaven and against you. I am no longer worthy to be called your son; make me like one of your hired servants."

So, he got up and went to his father. But while he was still a long way off, his father saw him and was filled with compassion for him; he ran to his son, threw his arms around him and kissed him. The son said to him, "Father, I have sinned against heaven and against you. I am no longer worthy to be called your son."

But the father said to his servants, "Quick! Bring the best robe and put it on him. Put a ring on his finger and sandals on his feet. Bring the fattened calf and kill it. Let's have a feast and celebrate. For this son of mine was dead and is alive again; he was lost and is found."

So, they began to celebrate. Meanwhile, the older son was in the field. When he came near the house, he heard music and dancing. So, he called one of the servants and asked him what was going on. "Your brother has come," he replied, "and your father has killed the fattened calf because he has him back safe and sound."

The older brother became angry and refused to go in. So, his father went out and pleaded with him. But he answered his father, "Look! All these years I've been slaving for you and never disobeyed your orders. Yet you never gave me even a young goat so I could celebrate with my friends. But when this son of yours who has squandered your property with prostitutes comes home, you kill the fattened calf for him!"

"My son," the father said, "you are always with me, and everything I have is yours. But we had to celebrate and be glad, because this brother of yours was dead and is alive again; he was lost and is found."[1]

He had no food, no job, and no home. He was at rock bottom with no options, but I love the next phrase in that story: "He came to his senses." The terrible part of pain is how much it hurts. The beautiful part is that it puts you in a position of having to think through a new approach. I was at the end of myself. I couldn't pray my way, sing my way, or read my way out of the hell of experiencing constant waves of panic. I was out of options. I needed a way out of the prison I had created. Like the lost son, I needed to run home to my Father. The pain forced me to pull the key to my prison out of my pocket and do the very thing that terrified me the most. On a bathroom floor in Keller, Texas, I finally said it out loud.

ENDNOTE

1. Luke 15:11-31.

CHAPTER THREE

LET ME OUT

I have a friend who used to yell from the stands to our girls' basketball team when it was time to play defense; "Pressure makes a pipe burst!" Everyone else would grin when he screamed it—I just thought about Friday.

Day Seventeen.

Day Seventeen was a Friday. It had been my favorite day of the week. The kids were at school. Friday was my day off, and we had decided early in our marriage to reserve that day for just the two of us. Sometimes we would go to the movies. Sometimes we would go to breakfast with friends. Sometimes we did projects around the house. I knew this Friday was going to be different than any of our date days, and it was definitely not one I had circled on the calendar. Mika was in the bathroom, putting on makeup and getting ready for the day. She was sitting in front of the mirror. I stood outside the door, rehearsing my speech, but I couldn't put two words together. Every time I would start the speech in my head, these movies filled with worst-case scenarios at the end of our conversation started going off in my imagination. I was terrified. I felt like I couldn't breathe. I stepped towards the door at least five times, but I just couldn't seem to put my hand on the knob and go in. It's hard to explain, but I felt like I was in the middle of a huge tug of war. Part of me had convinced myself that this would be the end of my marriage and it scared me to death. The other part of me believed that I didn't deserve a family like the one I had and I felt a weird sense of relief that I was finally going to get what I deserved. The pressure was building, and I was about to burst. Finally, I walked in, sat down on the floor beside Mika, took a deep breath, and said, "I need to tell you something."

Confession.

Jesus said, "Then you will know truth. And the truth will set you free."

James Garfield said, "The truth will set you free, but first it will make you miserable."

The truth was that I needed to be set free and I was miserable. Garfield's words may make you laugh just a little. Jesus's words, on the other hand, are powerful and poignant. The truth **will** set you free and the inverse of that principle is true as well. If the truth sets you free, then a lie will leave you living locked up and trapped. That's where I found myself that Friday. I was imprisoned by lies I had believed for a long time. It was as if they were on repeat in my head-playing over-and-over again. The lies were like bars I could not break or bend, and I just wanted someone to let me out.

You'll never be good enough.

You need to be perfect.

You will never measure up.

Your anxiety is punishment for your lack of faith.

You deserve the misery you are living in.

I had listened to these lies for so long they had become "my truth." Those truths are always the enemy of actual truth. The results of believing those lies across time was a deep sense of shame. Disappointed in myself, I was convinced that if people really knew my fears, my doubts, my struggles, they would want nothing to do with me. I was that little boy on the baseball field all over again. I was stuck in a cycle of wondering if God would think I was good enough and believing I could get control of all of this if I just tried harder. I was miserable and believed I deserved every ounce of guilt I felt for the condition I found myself in.

Full of shame.

Alone.

Isolated.

Let me out.

Shame convinces you that everything about you is flawed, and shame is not the same as guilt. Guilt is about something we have done. Shame does not distinguish bad behavior. Shame convinces us that we are bad. Shame is not about what we have done, it is about who we are. Shame says, "You are inadequate," and it overshadows and clouds every thought or emotion you have. It permeates your soul until it deteriorates your esteem. You withdraw from others, seeking solace in isolation, or at least protection from being exposed. Isolation is another tool of the enemy. In isolation, you wall yourself off from those who love you and can help you through your problems. It is cruel to be surrounded by help but convinced you are on your own and inadequate. Solitude is healthy, it allows you to clear the noise and connect with God. Isolation is brutally harmful, it drowns out the voice of God and causes you to disconnect from everyone.

We can isolate ourselves or we can be isolated because of consequences of our actions. Isolation in solitary confinement has been studied by scientists. According to *Psychology Today,* solitary confinement significantly impacts the brain. "Solitary confinement as a punishment is closer to a form of torture, with serious consequences for neurological health. Teams of researchers are investigating further the deep effects of this practice and studying the possibility of regulating it to maintain physical activity as well as sensory input and circadian rhythms, in order to prevent profound changes in the brain."[1]

Isolation affects you mentally as well as physically. It is a crushing environment where God never intended us to live. When you mix isolation with shame, you have a powerful and poisonous combination. Together, they erode your sense of worth and value and convince you that you are not deserving of love. They whisper to your soul, "You are not enough," and you begin to believe it to be true. Over time and in isolation long enough, you start having doubts about goods things. When something good happens to

WHEN YOU MIX
ISOLATION WITH
SHAME, YOU HAVE
A POWERFUL
AND POISONOUS
COMBINATION

you, you cannot trust that feeling. Instead of finding joy, you wait anxiously for the other shoe to drop. It's this constant state of dis-ease that torments your soul.

That's where I found myself that Friday. Trust me, coming clean about it to Mika wasn't an act of courage, it was desperation. I had run out of options. I knew I was at the bottom of a valley I had no chance of climbing out of alone. My heart was pounding, my palms were sweating, and I could feel the tension in every muscle as I worked up the courage to say,

"Mika, I'm in trouble.

"I think I'm going crazy.

"I don't know what to do ..."

Those words choked in my throat. Tears ran down my face, and more words spilled out of my mouth in a torrent. I told her all of my irrational fears. I opened up about all the negative thoughts I had been wrestling with—the shortcomings I felt as a husband, the inadequacies I felt as a father, my failings as a friend. I finally told her the whole truth about my inability to sleep or to control my breathing, and how terrifying it was the way my heart kept racing.

She listened without interruption, letting me spill it all out. Totally drained I managed to say at last, "I'm sorry for what I've become. You deserve better than this, you deserve better than me."

I was out of words.

I was out of tears.

I was out.

Let me out.

Exhausted, my head dropped to my chest. I sat there believing she would walk out the door. It's what I expected. It is what I felt like I deserved.

But she didn't walk out.

She didn't leave.

She stayed.

She gently raised my chin with her index finger. My swollen red eyes met the steady kindness in hers. In a soft yet strong voice full of grace, she whispered, "Toby, I don't know what this is, but we will get through this together. You are a good man, and I love you."

I shook my head, not daring to believe she could love me in my mess, but her eyes held my gaze. She kept talking to me. She prayed as she comforted me. She said a lot of things that day, most of which I don't remember exactly, but those two sentences are forever burned in my memory. Her two sentences contained unconditional love. It's impossible to forget an experience where you are overcome with unconditional love.

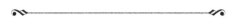

I grew up in a house with a yard that backed up to the local Catholic church. Many of my friends were a part of that parish. I would see their cars in the parking lot quite regularly on weekday afternoons. One day, I asked one of the girls I knew why her car was there every week on a day other than Sunday. "I go to confession," she told me.

As a boy growing up in the Church of Christ, I had no paradigm for the concept of confession. *You mean, sit in a booth and tell someone all of your mistakes every week? Why would anyone sign up for that?* I asked myself. But that Friday morning on a bathroom floor in Keller, Texas, I began to understand the power behind the principle of confession. Listen to the words of James, the brother of Jesus:

> *"... confess your sins to each other and pray for each other so*
> *that you may be healed ..."*[2]

The prison of shame and the punishment of isolation are created by the lie, "If I'm ever fully known, I'll never be fully loved." The real cruelty of this lie is that the very thing that can begin to release you is the thing which scares you the most. The truth is that I can never be fully loved until I am fully known. I can't experience unconditional love unless I put myself in the position of being loved without condition. Terrifying? Yes. Necessary? Definitely.

Speaking the truth about where you are, the fears you feel, and the lies you're having a hard time not believing is the key that begins to unlock your prison doors. I don't know who said it, but it's true: there's no healing in hiding. James said, confessing our sins to one another brings healing. Once again, the inverse of that principle is true. If confession brings you healing, then secrets make you sick.

Irrational fears seem very real when you're experiencing them. I was convinced Mika was going to leave me that day. That seems crazy now, but at that time, it did not, it felt like reality. Your challenge may be different than mine, but no matter what fears you are confronting, the progression is always the same.

- Fears are based on lies.
- Lies lead to shame.
- Shame leads to isolation.

- Isolation leads to prison.

- The only way to get out is to let somebody in.

- Say it out loud—confess—and watch shame lose its power—be healed.

- Fear loses its bite when it is out in the open.

- Darkness gets lighter … and so does your spirit.

As one who has been there, I encourage you to fight the urge to step back behind the prison walls. I know the urge is real because I've lived it. There are times when it is still more comfortable for me to put the key to my prison back in my pocket, paste a big smile on my face, and try to fool others into believing that I'm something or somewhere I'm not. That's an exhausting way to live. It will suck the life right out of you. I know, it almost took me out.

Almost every time I open up and share about anxiety and my battle with feeling "less than," someone contacts me and comments on my "brave authenticity." I appreciate their words, but for me, I don't see authenticity as bravery; I see it as my primary weapon in the battle for my heart. Speaking the truth to my wife, to my close relationships, and to my church family humbles me; and the One who created me gives grace to the humble. I need grace.

IN THE BATTLE FOR MY HEART, CONFESSION IS MY PRIMARY WEAPON

Confession is a weapon.

Confession brings healing.

Confession is good for my soul.

You are probably like me and feel like it's embarrassing to admit your fears. Admit them anyway. Well-intentioned people may try to fix the unfixable when you are honest about where you are. Say it out loud anyway. You won't always experience love without condition, and that hurts, but don't go back to shallow living. It may feel suitable for a moment, it may even feel like protection, but the end result is your soul locked up in a prison of your own making. Find a community where you can be fully known and fully loved. Experience the freedom that can only come when you have nothing to hide.

Be known.

Be loved.

Break free.

ENDNOTES

1. *The Effects of Solitary Confinement on the Brain* by Elana Blanco-Suarez, Ph.D. Posted 27 February, 2019. © *Psychology Today*. Retrieved on 05 November, 2019 at: https://www.psychologytoday.com/us/blog/brain-chemistry/201902/the-effects-solitary-confinement-the-brain.
2. James 5:16.

EXPERIENCE THE
FREEDOM THAT CAN
COME ONLY WHEN YOU
HAVE NOTHING TO HIDE

CHAPTER FOUR

WOUNDING THE WALKING

Approximately 40 million Americans struggle with an anxiety disorder, and about 2 percent of these individuals are prone to panic attacks. A panic attack is a sudden episode of intense fear that triggers severe physical reactions where you feel completely out of control and often feel like you're dying.

—MIKE FOSTER *FUN THERAPY PODCAST*

Honesty is the best policy. Yes, telling the truth is a better way to live; but sometimes it doesn't feel that way. It will make you miserable before it sets you free. There have been many times over the past twenty years that I have doubted my decision to share my battles with anxiety and panic publicly. I knew I needed to tell the truth about how I was struggling. I wanted my closest friends and my family to know what I was dealing with on a day to day basis, but fear kept me from revealing the truth. Even though I knew sharing would invite the ensuing result of feeling less than—inadequate, insufficient, weak … you get the idea. I would stand up and teach Sunday after Sunday about how Christ wants to meet you right where you are, that you should step out in faith, let Him meet you in your weaknesses, Christ is the only way you can find the power to overcome in the first place … but the truth—the cold hard truth—was that I was afraid. No, more than just afraid, I was also ashamed.

I was wrestling with an element of shame. Parts of my heart were struggling with questions about acceptance and fears regarding judgment from others. Anxiety came even when I was trusting God. It sometimes happened (and happens still) even when I am full of faith. And well-intended Christian friends insinuating that if I just prayed more, had more faith, believed in a bigger God, fill-in-the-blank … only made things worse.

I remember teaching about how Jesus wants to walk right into the middle of "that issue" in your life. I would tell myself over and over again that He's not waiting for me to get it all cleaned up first and that He wants to meet me in the middle of my mess and muck and pain. I knew this to be truth, but the advice pouring in from my Christian brothers and sisters made it tough to remember. In fact, my doubts and questions have almost always come from the responses and reactions I get from Jesus followers with their *Ten Steps to Overcome Anxiety*, *Daily Declarations for a Calm You* and a host of other quick and easy "Bible solutions" to resolve all my struggles. I can't begin to count the number of conversations, letters, or emails I've received over the years from men and women who say "they just want to help" but their "help" is to offer a plethora of performance rituals for me to follow—opportunities for me to ***do better***. Most of the time,

Jesus gives me enough grace to smile and nod, hit delete, or practice my jump shot into the nearest wastebasket.

On February 9, 2017, however, my patience ran out. My emotions took over. I was working at home, trying to empty my inbox. I opened an email and read it, the too-familiar "help" message struck a nerve. I closed my eyes and took a deep breath. Like many times in the past, I deleted it instantly. But this time, on this day, I opened Facebook and started to pound the keys. Today I needed to respond.

Dear Well-Intentioned, Jesus-Loving, Bible-Believing Friend,

I say this with all the love I can muster—I really do: you're not helping. I know you want to, but you're not. In fact, you're hurting. I know you don't mean to, but you really are. I hate conflict and confrontation is not my thing, but I have to say something, so here goes:

Anxiety and worry are two different things. Worry happens when I let small things get big, when I try to control outcomes that are outside of my control. Jesus invites us (or commands us if that's the way you see Scripture—but that's for another letter) to release our worry to Him, to recognize that outcomes are His deal and not ours. Opening up His Book and reading His truth about who He is and who I am helps me to move out of the worry cycle. Connecting with Him (who lives inside of me already) through prayer takes my focus from my issues to His greatness. Worship, declaring the truth of who He is, releases supernatural power and brings an unexplainable lifting of my spirit and my soul. Jesus offers me all of these things as my Shepherd and my Source, and they are good and helpful and life-giving.

Anxiety is not worrying. Anxiety is about my decision to try to control things outside of my control. Anxiety is waking up at 3:00 in the morning with heart pounding, drenched in sweat, breathing as if I just finished a 400-meter dash. Anxiety is the debilitating feeling that everything is spinning out of control for no apparent reason. Anxiety attacks come unexpectedly. Sometimes they come when I'm really tired, spiritually depleted, or in a season of activity and stress. But sometimes they come FOR NO REASON AT ALL. They come when I'm rested, when my heart and my mind are full, when my soul is connected to Him. Honestly, there's no rhyme or reason to it in my life, and trust me, I've spent hours trying to figure it out. Anxiety challenges my manhood and my faith. It causes me to doubt myself, and when the attacks come for an extended period, begin to question even the only Source I have to get me through the nightmare of those seasons.

So, I'm asking with everything I have in me, please stop taking the invitation of Jesus not to worry and applying it to my battle with anxiety and panic. Telling me to "pray more" or "believe bigger" or "get in the Word" actually makes my battle worse. It plants the seed that if somehow, I could just be better or do better, I wouldn't have these challenges. It makes me feel "less than" in so many ways. You wouldn't tell your diabetic friend that there was some formula for their healing, would you? You would never (even unintentionally) lead them to believe that they were sick because of a lack of faith or spirituality? I know you wouldn't! I know that's not your heart. You love me, and you want the best for me. Pray for me. Ask God to do what I haven't been able to do. Be patient with me. I just thought you'd want to know.[1]

I hit the share button.

I will admit, I was emotionally charged up. I had some things that I had wanted to say for a long time and up until that moment, had always decided not to. I don't recommend ever posting about anything if you find yourself fired up. It's rarely a good idea, but that afternoon, I decided it was time for me to draw a circle around all those walking in their woundedness. I closed my computer and went on with my day.

A friend texted me a few hours later and asked if I had seen what was happening on my Facebook page. I opened up my computer, logged on to my page, and quietly stared at the number of people who had begun to share my little rant with their friends. Over the next couple of days, I spent time just reading the comments from all over the country from people who basically said in some form or fashion, "Thanks for writing what I've been feeling."

"... I too suffer from anxiety and am having a rough go of it right now. I have trouble verbalizing what it feels like to be going through this, so I shared this post with my husband

to help him better understand. Thank you for being so real
and transparent ...!"   —Natalie B.

"You just expressed everything I always thought but could
never get out. As someone that suffered from anxiety
attacks for a long time, I appreciate this so much ..."
                                                —Sara L.

It broke my heart.

The situations were varied, but the story was the same. Wounded people who should be finding hope, grace, encouragement, and life from their communities of faith were receiving NONE of those things. Their words described things like feeling judged, condemned, shamed, and embarrassed. They went in feeling less than, and they were leaving feeling less than less than.

We've got to do a better job in this area. You and me. All of us. We need to be extremely sensitive to the fact that sometimes what seems to be helping is actually hurting. The church's view on mental illness and issues related to emotional health needs some refinement. We don't tell a person with diabetes to pray harder, have more faith, skip your insulin and declare your body to produce its own. Our compassion and concern for physical health should be congruent with our compassion and concern for emotional health. We believe God can fully heal all things, but we leave issues involving mental

> OUR COMPASSION AND CONCERN FOR PHYSICAL HEALTH SHOULD BE CONGRUENT WITH OUR COMPASSION AND CONCERN FOR EMOTIONAL HEALTH

illness in a category all to itself. I have prayed for people who believe God has healed them from their battle. I have faith that He has moved mountains in people's lives regarding panic and anxiety. I have seen physical healings that have taken my breath away. Though I believe God is totally capable of healing me from them, panic and anxiety are part of my everyday life. This is still my limp, my thorn, my battle. And I think we, as Christians, can do better. We are called to do better.

Paul says,

> Therefore, there is now **no condemnation** for those who are in Christ Jesus, because through Christ Jesus the law of the Spirit who gives life has set you free from the law of sin and death.[2]

No condemnation.

No **condemnation**.

Reread it …

No condemnation.

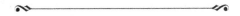

So, what do we do? How do we walk alongside others who struggle with panic and anxiety? Here are a few things we can do to keep from wounding the walking:

- **Be quiet—just listen.** Some of the best relationship advice ever written is found in the book of James: "Be quick to listen and slow to speak."[3] This applies in a myriad of contexts, but it is especially applicable to this discussion. Many times, the need to say something compels us into using phrases and terms that hurt the very hearts we want to help. Not having an answer is not a sign of weakness or lack of spiritual strength. Sometimes the words, "I'm sorry," and "I'm here" mean more than some religious formula or catchphrase. Release yourself from the need to have all of the answers and love people right where they are. Be quiet—just listen.

- **Love**. That's enough. Religion is all about performance. Religion is quick to tell someone what to do. Jesus is all about love—radical, unconditional, hope-giving love. If you've surrendered your life the best way that you know how to the love of Jesus, then He lives in you. Make sure your response to the people around you who are struggling has a whole lot of Jesus and avoids religion at all costs. Folks who feel less than need to experience the One who is greater than. No matter where we live or what we do for a living—this is our destiny. We were created by God to be a bridge to His love, grace, and transforming power. Let's stop being a barrier to people finding the very thing that their heart longs for.

- **Speak like Jesus**. Let's be known as people who believe the best about people and for people. We all walk with a limp. Every one of us fights battles at some level that cause us to question our worth and value. If you're breathing, you've been in that battle. Telling someone who they are is so much better than telling someone what they should do. Your words have power—speak life and not death. It's the way of Jesus.

I have felt judged. I have felt looked down on. There have been seasons where it seemed as if everyone was trying to fix me. I have been on my knees, quoting scripture—literally surrounding myself with scripture written down on cards. I am in the process of overcoming every single day, but even fully surrendered to Jesus and His changing power, I cannot say this is behind me. I feel a special kinship with those who walk with a limp and don't quite have a pretty bow at the end of their story. They are living in the *Not Yet*.

Let's not forget that we are all learning. We are all in process. What we need to remember most of all is that we cannot do this by ourselves. We were not intended to fight our battles alone. We need to surround ourselves with people who will walk with us, and we need to be a people who deeply desire God's best for us and who will stand in the gaps for us when we are struggling. We need to release ourselves from believing that we have to impress people. In the past, I have cared way too much about what others have thought of me. This hindered my ability to engage with the truth. Now, I continually remind myself of John's words:

> *Then you will **know the truth**, and the truth **will set you free**.*[4]

ENDNOTES

1. https://www.facebook.com/tobyslough/posts/1441386765880916?__
   tn__=K-R. Note: Some minor edits were made to this post for grammar
   (since we had the opportunity), but this excerpt is the real, raw,
   unfiltered letter Toby shared with the world on 19 February, 2017.

2. Romans 8:1-2 (author emphasis).

3. James 1:19.

4. John 8:32 (author emphasis).

THOSE WHO FEEL "LESS
THAN" ARE IN THE MOST
NEED OF EXPERIENCING THE
ONE WHO IS "GREATER THAN"

CHAPTER FIVE

FIX ME

Three times, I pleaded with the Lord

to take it away from me.[1]

—PAUL

Do you remember Saturday morning cartoon shows? When I was a kid, we didn't have streaming, and we certainly couldn't binge-watch. I know I risk dating myself by even bringing this up, but we could only watch a show when the television station actually aired it. This made Saturday mornings a much-anticipated weekly event! I would wake up early to watch *Looney Tunes®*. The simplistic storylines entertained me, made me laugh, caused me to me smile, and gave me something to look forward to each weekend. I had a whole host of favorite characters, and I am sure you had a favorite or two yourself.

Of the Wile E. Coyote and Road Runner duo, Road Runner was my favorite, although I must admit to having a bit of a love/hate relationship with him. Wile E., better known simply as Coyote, was always chasing Road Runner out in the hot, dusty desert where they lived. Though Coyote was never able to catch Road Runner, he always seemed to figure out a way to order some contraption from the Acme Company that was delivered right when he needed it! I would rush to my favorite spot on our couch in the living room as the theme song would start to play:

> *If you're on a highway and Road Runner goes beep beep.*
> *Just step aside, or you might end up in a heap.*
> *Road Runner, Road Runner, runs down the road all day.*
> *Even the coyote can't make him change his ways.*
>
> *Road Runner, the coyote's after you.*
> *Road Runner, if he catches you, you're through.*
> *Road Runner, the coyote's after you.*
> *Road Runner, if he catches you, you're through.*
>
> *That coyote is really a crazy clown,*
> *When will he learn that he never can mow him down?*
> *Poor little Road Runner never bothers anyone,*
> *Just runnin' down the road's his idea of having fun.*[2]

If you are old enough to remember watching this cartoon, you are welcome for that earworm—you'll now be singing it all day! Who doesn't love the Road Runner?! He was crafty, shifty, speedy, a bit of a know-it-all, but for the most part, a likable bird. Road Runner was the arch-nemesis of Wile E. Coyote whose ingenuity and assortment of Acme products like glue, grease, gigantic rubber bands, anvils, and of course, dynamite was always impressive. Wile E. tried scheme after scheme to catch Road Runner, but he never found just the right formula. I always believed for Coyote's victory. Often, I found the chase to be very frustrating. I kept waiting for one of the Coyote's devices to work, but the Road Runner always found a way to turn the trap around and use it to his own advantage. I loved that the Road Runner was such a great escape artist, but I secretly wanted him to get caught at least once! One Saturday after another, the chase continued.

Will he ever catch what he's chasing? I'd ask myself at the end of every episode.

Sitting on the couch as a small boy, I couldn't see what would be waiting for me several miles up the road. I stared at the television blissfully unaware that one day, like Road Runner, I would find myself in the chase for my life. I had a few decades before my chase would begin, and just like Wile E. Coyote, I too would be getting an anvil dropped on my head at every turn.

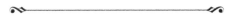

It was in my early thirties that I first began to experience panic attacks. In the beginning, I wasn't sure what to call them. Most times, I had no idea what was happening. Since I didn't know what was happening, I had no clue as to how to avoid them. Day after day, I would experience them, and I had no idea how to make them stop. I would physically recover after each of them, but I would be completely exhausted. Spent, tired, and frustrated, the panic attacks were consuming my physical, mental, and emotional energy. I would tell myself over and over again that I was going to be alright. I would say to myself, *I can get through this. Hang on.* This was not in my imagination, the panic attacks were real. Their effects on my life began to pile up, weighing me down, breaking my spirit. The consistent wave upon wave of anxiety attacks, sleeplessness, nausea, vomiting, and inability to find any relief broke me. Just reading these words makes me feel it in my chest. It was at that low point that I decided I needed to get professional help. I knew I needed to find a counselor who could help me. Being a pastor, my pride wouldn't allow me to see anyone in a church setting. That is hard to admit, but there were certain circumstances and specific pressures that led me to squelch my authenticity. Some of those were self-inflicted beliefs and may or may not have been accurate. I wrestled with thoughts like:

What would I do if someone from the church saw me?

What would they think of me if anyone found out about this?

Would the elders ask me to step down if they knew how badly I was struggling?

How can I help other people with their lives if my own life is falling apart?

My wife, Mika, and I began our search for a "Christian counselor" in a phone book (which also dates me). We found one, and thankfully, he was on the other side of the city. I thought that was a perfect solution. Having him on the opposite side of where I worked and lived seemed like a workable situation. It would be that much easier for me to keep my secret—my secret that I had hit rock bottom. I had settled into the unsettling rhythm of fear, lack of self-worth, extreme fatigue, and loss of appetite. *At least I can't go any lower,* I thought. I was sure I was at rock bottom.

I drove myself across town to my counselor's building. Nervously, I made my way to the office door. It took so much courage for me to grab the doorknob and move across that canyon of a threshold. I was unsteady at best. It was a moment of total desperation. I walked into the counselor's office, greeted him with an impish smile, sunk deep into his overstuffed chair and said, "I think I'm going crazy. You don't know me. I'm at the end of me. I'll do whatever you ask, but you have just to fix me."

He smiled knowingly, then drew in an easy breath and began to ask questions. I could tell the questions were structured to assess my current state of mind. I knew the truthful answers to what he was asking, yet it took me less than two minutes to tell my first lie. He asked if I had ever considered hurting myself, and I dishonestly and firmly said, "No." I also let him know that I didn't want to waste my time or money talking about my childhood years or whether or not my mom had diapered me correctly.

"I just want you to make this go away," I told him.

I went three days a week for the first couple of weeks. If you have spent any time in counseling, and I hope you have, you know that three times per week outside of a clinical setting is a lot. My counselor and I had initial discussions centered around coping techniques that I should use when I felt a panic attack coming on. He needed to get me to a place where I could deal, where I could function, where I could manage. There were specific actions I would repeat, certain words I would say, etc. that would help me get to a place where I could handle getting to the root of things. At this point in the chase, anything was better than what I was experiencing. I found myself living from appointment to appointment, using the "pop a rubber band on my wrist" technique, or practicing breathing techniques when the black wave of anxiety started rolling over me. Anytime my counselor tried to ask a question that could potentially take me beyond my threshold of comfort, I would shut down. A literal shut down, like backed up traffic on I-35. This shut down was something I could feel in every cell of my body. Even with his gracious manner of gently waking me up to those dark places, I couldn't go there. I couldn't get to the root of the root. I needed to develop the muscles for coping that would help me chase down my roadrunner. It was the only thing that could help me work my way through the dark. I was miles into the chase, and this time, I was Road Runner, and Wile E. was hot on my tail.

During the third week of this chase, things got real. It began with an innocent start to what seemed to be the beginnings of a regular session. A simple question was posed from my new friend, the counselor,

"How many panic attacks could you have a week and still be okay?"

"None. Zero." was my instant and emphatic reply.

"Okay, how many in a month?" was the next question, and my response was the same.

"None. Zero."

This went on for over ten minutes until I responded to his "How many in a year?" question with the same level of intensity and passion (stubbornness) as I had when the questioning began.

"**None. Zero.**"

"Are you telling me that you cannot be happy, at peace, or satisfied if you had even one panic attack in a year?" he asked, an incredulous look was on his face.

I looked him straight in the eye and replied straight away, "God is a Healer, and I know that He will heal me. I will never be satisfied with anything less than His best for me. There is an answer, and I will find it," I told him.

None.

Zero.

We worked together week after week. As we worked, I prayed for complete healing. I fully believed God would heal me. I faithfully practiced my techniques and my newly learned coping skills. I saw this counselor for several months. I was amazed at the amount of patience this man had for me and with me. We made gains, and even though we had come a long way together, I knew we had miles of work ahead of us. My goal was to eliminate panic attacks from my life completely, and I was determined to work tenaciously to make that happen. I had faith in this man, and throughout our time together, had grown to trust him with this most painful part of my life. I deeply desired to be the best husband, father, pastor, and friend I could be. I was willing to do the hard work to get myself back on track, my life back to normal, my health back to what it once was.

MY GOAL WAS TO ELIMINATE PANIC ATTACKS FROM MY LIFE COMPLETELY

Then one day, my counselor walked into one of our church services. It was obviously strange to see him in my environment. I went up to him, said hello, and told him it was good to see him. His eyes were locked in a gaze at his shoes. This time, he was the one who looked unsteady. His hands were nervously hidden in his pocket. His presence was much like mine had been in that overstuffed chair—awkward, uncomfortable, and unsettled. This time, I could see he was the one mustering courage and grappling for words. Sheepishly, he shared some devastating news. He had come to say goodbye. His marriage had blown up, and he was moving back to the East coast.

I went home that night and cried.

Now, what am I going to do?

My desperation turned to determination. I have always been a competitor. You name the sport, the game, the contest and I will work tirelessly hard to win. I was sure that if I just did a gut check, I could muscle my way to victory over this, the ultimatum I had given God in my heart that day—the total absence of any anxiety or panic—led me on the chase of a lifetime. I wasn't going to lose.

None.

Zero.

I was convinced there was "an answer" out there—I had just to find IT. The IT was out there, and I was going to chase it down. Maybe worship music was the answer. I had it going day and night. I read books on prayer and convinced myself that if I just learned to "pray better," God would give me what I wanted. I read the Psalms over and over. I started going to every charismatic gathering that promoted any type of healing service. If the event had the word fire, blood, or victory in it, I was there. In healing services, I stepped forward every time the band started playing the music for the altar call. I've had more oil poured on my head than a car with a leaky valve at Jiffy Lube. People hit the ground as eloquent, passionate speakers raised their hands and declared healing and victory. But not me. I was always left standing, wondering what they were getting that I was not. Week after week, I was left standing. But I was not giving up.

None.

Zero.

"Jesus didn't die for you to battle anxiety," became my battle cry. I was chasing healing as hard as I could, as often as I could. There would be moments where I would convince myself that the cloud had been lifted, and I would declare myself healed. But the black wave would come again and again.

I battled with song. I battled with prayer. I battled with scripture:

> *Three times, I pleaded with the Lord to take it away from me. But he said to me, "My grace is sufficient for you, for my power is made perfect in weakness." Therefore, I will boast all the more gladly about my weaknesses, so that Christ's power may rest on me. That is why, for Christ's sake, I delight in weaknesses, in insults, in hardships, in persecutions, in difficulties. For when I am weak, then I am strong.*[3]

I don't know if Paul literally asked God for healing three times or if he asked God for healing three hundred times. I don't know if his requests came over weeks or months. I don't know if those requests came year after year. I'm not exactly sure and neither are Bible scholars in agreement as to what Paul was seeking regarding his healing. What I do know is that I could relate to Paul's pleads to God. I refused to give up on my healing as I begged like Paul.

Eighteen months after my first anxiety attack, I found myself in my second counselor's office. This was a completely different experience than my first one. At this point, I was struggling to find the words to describe how I was feeling. I was weary in every sense of the word. I was tired of people giving me verses on worry. I took their offer of verse after verse on how to offset worry as off-putting. I felt like they were basically telling me to stop sinning.

I was slowly losing the chase. I was losing my grip on rational thoughts. Dangerous places of unhealthiness were gaining ground in my life taking their seat in dark corners of my heart that saw little to no light. I had this desperate and very unhealthy desire for Mika to "get it." I wanted her to understand my pain, grasp my struggle, to comprehend the chase even though I couldn't find the words to describe any of it to her adequately.

My second counselor helped me put words to what I was experiencing. I found this to be very helpful when trying to explain what I was going through to my very small circle of trusted friends. The definition he gave me in my first session has stuck with me all these years. "If you're house burned down and six months later you find yourself at a stoplight, and a fire truck comes up behind you, your heart will automatically begin to race, that is normal," he said. "But if you've never experienced a fire and your heart begins to race, and you become convinced that the fire truck is headed to your house, and you can't shake that feeling—that's an anxiety problem."

Wherever I turned, whatever I did, my life was a chase filled with irrational fears screaming from fire trucks at stoplights. With tears streaming down my face, I pleaded with him, "Can you please help me?"

The weeks that followed were more complicated and more frustrating than I could have ever imagined. Life in the rearview mirror is so much clearer. I can see now how God was intentionally working to peel back layers of my heart. He knew exactly what my heart could take and what it couldn't. But I sure couldn't see it then. This counselor refused to talk about coping techniques. He gently reminded me that those things were dealing with symptoms, and he was trying to get to the heart of the problem. He kept asking me about my growing up years, and when I wanted to shut him down, he would just sit there and look at me.

One day we spent over fifty minutes of a ninety-minute session just looking at each other. Over time, I realized my struggle to recognize deficiencies in my relationship with my dad was based upon my desire to be an honoring son. I came to understand that the simple recognition of anything less than perfection was not helpful or healthy for him or for me.

The Lord used this man to help me understand that anything I didn't get from my father was because he hadn't gotten it from his, and it was possible to recognize it, forgive it, and live with honor and love. He never "declared me healed," but I'll always remember our last time together. As we knelt together to pray, the distinct sound of a siren filled the air. We laughed, I wept and went home believing deep in my heart for the first time that God was with me—He hadn't left me, and He still heard my cries for help. Someone had opened a window, and I was finally beginning to see a little light at the end of the tunnel. The chase wasn't over, but for the first time, I didn't feel so alone.

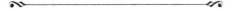

Chasing isn't always a bad thing, it's just exhausting when you chase the wrong thing. In my version of the Bible, it's called "seeking." As I look back, my problem wasn't that I was chasing something, my problem was the something I was chasing. David talks about seeking God's face—His Presence. I was seeking (read that chasing) His hand—His blessing. Asking God to bless you is a good thing. Believing that you need to chase God because you haven't received what you're asking for is life-sucking, because, the fact of the matter is, God is always there.

The Lord is my light and my salvation—whom shall, I fear?

The Lord is the stronghold of my life—
of whom shall I be afraid?

When the wicked advance against me to devour me,
it is my enemies and my foes who will stumble and fall?

Though an army besiege me, my heart will not fear;
though war break out against me,
even then I will be confident.

One thing I ask from the Lord, this only do I seek:
that I may dwell in the house of the
Lord all the days of my life,
to gaze on the beauty of the Lord and
to seek him in his temple.

For in the day of trouble he will keep
me safe in his dwelling;
he will hide me in the shelter of his sacred
tent and set me high upon a rock.

Then my head will be exalted above
the enemies who surround me;
at his sacred tent I will sacrifice with shouts of joy;

I will sing and make music to the Lord.

Hear my voice when I call, Lord; be
merciful to me and answer me.

My heart says of you, "Seek his face!"

Your face, Lord, I will seek.

Do not hide your face from me,
do not turn your servant away in anger;
you have been my helper.

Do not reject me or forsake me,

God my Savior.

Though my father and mother forsake me,
the Lord will receive me.

Teach me your way, Lord;
lead me in a straight path because of my oppressors.

Do not turn me over to the desire of my foes,
for false witnesses rise up against me,
spouting malicious accusations.

I remain confident of this:

I will see the goodness of the Lord in the land of the living.

Wait for the Lord;
be strong and take heart and wait for the Lord.[4]

My relationship with God was based on what He could do for me, not who He is. Pain does that sometimes. It causes us to issue ultimatums and define blessing. And it sets us up for disappointment. I'll never forget the night I sensed the Lord asking me, "Am I enough for you?" and the realization that my honest answer was "No—I need you to take this away, and then that will be enough." I was hoping for *something* and not in *Someone*.

My relationship with God had become dysfunctional. I was beginning to realize that my problem was not THE problem. Comprehending this was the first step on a long journey toward the life I had been looking for. I had a long way to go (and still do), but the afternoon I heard the siren, something began to shift.

With such relief, I thought that moment signaled the end of a painful season. I did not yet know that the journey towards freedom had just begun.

ENDNOTES

1.   2 Corinthians 12:8.
2.   Road Runner Theme Lyrics. http://www.lyricsondemand. com. Retrieved 07 November, 2019.
3.   2 Corinthians 12:8-10.
4.   Psalm 27.

CHAPTER SIX

UNFORCED RHYTHMS OF GRACE

Are you tired? Worn out? Burned out on religion? Come to me. Get away with me and you'll recover your life. I'll show you how to take a real rest. Walk with me and work with me—watch how I do it. **Learn the unforced rhythms of grace.** *I won't lay anything heavy or ill-fitting on you. Keep company with me and you'll learn to live freely and lightly.*

—MATTHEW 11:28-30, MSG

Categories make us comfortable. We like being able to define people, problems, behaviors, and outcomes clearly. If we can mentally fit something into a particular box, then maybe (we think), we can make sense of it all, and ultimately find a solution. The problem with this line of thinking is that everything doesn't always fit into neat columns. You have a mind, a body, and a spirit. Stress, pain, or pressure in one area of your being almost always affects another aspect of who you are. Freedom in one area does not necessarily equate to freedom in every area. There is the reality of both the natural and the supernatural, and they are intrinsically connected.

Many people ask me if I think my battle with anxiety is physical, emotional, or spiritual. My answer to that question is, "Yes." I have become acutely aware of how connected my mind, soul, and body are and the futility of trying to compartmentalize any challenge in my life into any one category. My spirit is affected by the focus of my mind. It's why when I'm asked to join friends at some blockbuster movie that is high in intensity or (God forbid) horror, I always decline. My standard answer is, "Thanks, I'm sure it will be great for you, but my heart beats fast regularly, I don't need to pay ten bucks to be scared." My physical condition affects and is affected by the level of my emotional health. If you have ever caught yourself stress eating, you know what I'm talking about!

Paul reminds me in Ephesians 6 of the reality of spiritual warfare. I don't pretend to understand it all, but I do know that there is an aspect of the battle that can only be won in the realm of the Spirit. Will power and self-help techniques are not enough. I need people praying for me, and I need to be connected to an ability beyond myself to live free. My soul has an enemy, and my body has serotonin levels. These two realities are connected because my spirit, soul, and body cannot be lumped into a single category.

My goal is to be healthy—whole—spiritually, physically, and emotionally. Though I have read much about the importance of balance, I have found that rhythm is a better concept for me. Life does not lend itself to balance. It is filled with seasons and cycles which will require more energy and attention to different things at different times. For me, balance is not sustainable. But I do need regular, consistent rhythms that nurture my heart, minister to my mind and feed my soul.

WORSHIP MUSIC

Certain songs stick in our heads for years for some reason. My now two-year-old grandkids couldn't tell you what they were doing ten minutes ago, but they can sing all the words to the theme song for "PJ Masks." Our connection to music is beyond sensory and greater than mere memory—music stirs the soul. You can hear a song after a decade of dormancy, and it will instantly transport you to another time and place.

I want to use that power of music to remember truths about God that will bring me life and hope. Knowing God's true character and nature is vital to a life of freedom. Until I know who He is, I will never fully grasp who He made me to be. My car radio is not always tuned to "Christian music" (sometimes a man needs a little Chris Stapleton or Beyoncé in his life!), but I make sure to regularly spend a portion of my forty-five-minute commute listening to a playlist with songs like:

- *Good, Good Father*
- *What A Beautiful Name*
- *Great Are You Lord*
- *How Great Thou Art*
- *Isn't He*
- *Waymaker*
- *Surrounded (Fight My Battles)*
- *New Wine*

I hear people talk about "ushering in God's presence." At one level, I understand what they are saying. I have been in church services where there is no doubt that His presence is filling the room. But I spent too many years of my life trying to invite God's presence into my car, my house, my office. Those moments in my car aren't about me ushering in God's presence—they are about the Spirit of God that lives in me being released into my head and my heart and replacing the lies that I can't seem to overcome. It is about me acknowledging His presence and coming into agreement with Him.

CONFESSION

If you grew up in church, the word confession probably has some negative vibes attached to it for you. You hear the word and think of walking to the front of a church building and telling someone some mistake you've made. Confession is all about sharing negative information with someone else. But in the Bible, the word confession literally means "to agree with God." Sometimes agreement with God is about acknowledging mistakes, but many times, agreement is about breaking mental images or patterns (the church word is "strongholds") that are making you feel less than and holding you back from the freedom you were created for. Health for me is, at its core, the regular practice of agreeing with God about who He is and who I am.

THE 40 I AMS

Several years ago, I found myself sitting in seat 1A on the anxiety bus. Desperate for relief, I called an older pastor friend and asked for help. He told me to Google "The 40 I AMs," print a copy, go in my closet, and begin to speak these words out loud. I quickly found them online and grabbed some index cards and began to handwrite the declaration and the verse for each one. An hour later, I finished, walked out in my backyard, sat down at our picnic table, and started reading the cards out loud. At first, I felt a bit awkward talking to myself in my back yard, but one day turned into two, and two turned into three, and before I knew it, I had gone three weeks without missing a day.

Confessing the Forty I Ams daily will cause you to see yourself the way God sees you. When you begin to see yourself from God's perspective, the opinions of others don't offend you. You are who God says you are.

1. A child of God. *Romans 8:16*

2. Redeemed from the hand of the enemy. *Psalms 107:2*

3. Forgiven. *Colossians 1:13-14*

4. Saved by grace through faith. *Ephesians 2:8*

5. Justified. *Romans 5:1*

6. Sanctified. *1 Corinthians 1:2*

7. A new creature. *2 Corinthians 5:17*

8. Partaker of His divine nature. *2 Peter 1:4*

9. Redeemed from the curse of the law. *Galatians 3:13*

10. Delivered from the powers of darkness. *Colossians 1:13*

11. Led by the Spirit of God. *Romans 8:14*

12. A son of God. *Romans 8:14*

13. Kept in safety wherever I go. *Psalms 91:11*

14. Getting all my needs met by Jesus. *Philippians 4:19*

15. Casting all my cares on Jesus. *1 Peter 5:7*

16. Strong in the Lord and in the power
    of His might. *Ephesians 6:10*

17. Doing all things through Christ who strengthens me. *Philippians 4:13*

18. An heir of God and a joint heir with Jesus. *Romans 8:17*

19. An heir to the blessing of Abraham. *Galatians 3:13-14*

20. Observing and doing the Lord's Commandments. *Deuteronomy 28:12*

21. Blessed coming in and blessed going out. *Deuteronomy 28:6*

22. An heir of eternal life. *1 John 5:11-12*

23. Blessed with all spiritual blessings. *Ephesians 1:3*

24. Healed by His stripes. *1 Peter 2:24*

25. Exercising my authority over the enemy. *Luke 10:19*

26. Above only and not beneath. *Deuteronomy 28:13*

27. More than a conqueror. *Romans 8:37*

28. Establishing God's Word here on earth. *Matthew 16:19*

29. An overcomer by the blood of the Lamb and the word of my testimony. *Revelation 12:11*

30. Daily overcoming the devil. *1 John 4:4*

31. Not moved by what I see. *2 Corinthians 4:18*

32. Walking by faith and not by sight. *2 Corinthians 5:7*

33. Casting down vain imaginations. *2 Corinthians 10:4-5*

34. Bringing every thought into captivity. *2 Corinthians 10:5*

35. Being transformed by renewing my mind. *Romans 12:1-2*

36. A laborer together with God. *1 Corinthians 3:9*

37. The righteousness of God in Christ. *2 Corinthians 5:21*

38. An imitator of Jesus. *Ephesians 5:1*

39. The light of the world. *Matthew 5:14*

40. Blessing the Lord at all times and continually praising Him with my mouth. *Psalms 34:1*

I didn't grow up in a religious tradition of liturgy, but this practice taught me about the beauty and potential of this rhythm in my life. Our faith is verbal in nature—it's why Jesus spoke, "Peace be still" on a stormy night on the Sea of Galilee. He could have just raised his hands or blinked his eyes, but He spoke it to show us the power of our words. His Father spoke the world into existence, He calmed a body of water with His words, and our words have the potential to change the atmosphere in us.

Thinking on the truths of who God says I am is good. Saying them aloud is better. I still carry those cards with me everywhere I go. They're in pretty bad shape—some of them are smeared with tears, others are covered in dirt and who knows what. I've pulled them out in some of my darkest moments and said the very words I'm having the hardest time believing—and God meets me there. I've thrown them on the ground in anger, shouting them like a crazy man, wondering where God is and if He is there at all. I have tried to figure out why He won't move them from my head to my heart. Even in the best of times, I try not to let a week go by without pulling them out and declaring the truth of who He says I am. The rhythm of it all has proven to be really good for my soul.

THE BEAUTIFUL RHYTHM OF LITERGY HAS PROVEN TO BE REALLY GOOD FOR MY SOUL

EXERCISE

Because I am so connected mind, body, and spirit, I have found some form of exercise to be vital to my emotional and spiritual health. We began in the Garden—created to be outside and active, and when our days consist of air conditioning and computer screens, it affects our heart and soul. Many times, in this area, we tend to think, "I can't do everything," and so we end up doing nothing. I can't always go to the gym for an hour, but I can always take a 15-minute walk. Exercise reduces stress, combats fatigue, improves alertness, and boosts concentration. I know that when I find time to jump on an elliptical when the weather is bad or take a power walk when the weather is good, I feel better. Better is good.

REST

If panic and worry have become your familiar routine, the concept of real rest is probably pretty foreign to you. The Bible says, *"An anxious heart weighs a man down."*[1] A heart weighed down is not at rest because it bears a burden. How then, if you are in the habit of carrying a burden, can you switch to a lifestyle of rest?

Jesus had such compassion for the heavy heart. He wants to take your burden and exchange it for rest. *"Come to me, all of you who are weary and carry heavy burdens, and I will give you rest. Take my yoke upon you. Let me teach you because I am humble and gentle, and you will find rest for your souls."*[2] Only the One who was fully God and fully man could make such an offer. Having walked the earth, Jesus was familiar with the burdensome struggles we face. However, as Creator of all things, He had the power to take those burdens and make them light for us. What an awesome and loving God!

Throughout his life, King David's burdens were many—fleeing a powerful king who wanted to kill him, running an entire nation, fighting nations much more substantial than his, and falling into tremendous sin. Complicated circumstances have surrounded him but listen to his testimony; *"When doubts filled my mind, your comfort gave me renewed hope and cheer."* [3] Not only did David release control of these situations, but he allowed God to bring him comfort.

Real rest is one of God's most precious gifts because it is one only He can give. Only He has the power to satisfy and sustain us. Only He knows me well enough to minister to my soul so directly. He brings me things no human has been or ever will be equipped to bring to me. When I go to Him for help and comfort, He never disappoints me. *"Cast all your anxiety on Him, because He cares for you."* [4]

Ridding yourself of the illusion that you can and should have control in life releases you from the deception that keeps you continually bound in anxiety. God's dream for you is that you would learn to trust His ultimate control, but His dream for you doesn't stop there! Jesus came not only to carry your burdens, but also give you rest from your weariness.

Remember the prodigal son? Once he realized that he had failed on his own, he decided the smartest thing to do would be to go back to his father. Life could only get better than living with the pigs. So, even if he could only work as a servant in his father's house, things would still be better than they were. Now, he was right in giving up his senseless way of life to return to the father, but it was apparent he didn't understand his father's heart. What happened when he returned and offered himself as a servant to his father? Did his father put him to work trading one burden for another? No, his father threw him a party and restored him as his son. He found rest.

Your Father wants to do the same for you! Once you decide to relinquish that control to Him, you shouldn't expect to live the rest of your life as a second-rate child in His family. He wants to give you fullness in Him and restore you entirely, even to the point where you find rest again.

SABBATH

Very early in the recorded history of God's people, God gave them "the big ten"—the Ten Commandments. Now, we know the ones about not murdering, not stealing, and not coveting. In fact, most of those moral laws are the foundation for our American laws. But many times, we pass over one of the commandments.

> *"Observe the Sabbath Day, to keep it holy. Work six days and do everything you need to do. But the seventh day is a Sabbath to God your God."*[5]

Listen to what God says as He is going to build His nation out of these people: *"Don't do any work, not you, nor your son, nor your daughter, nor your servant, nor your maid, nor your animals. Not even the foreign guests visiting in your town. For in six days God made heaven, earth and sea, and everything in them. He rested on the seventh day. Therefore, God blessed the Sabbath Day. He set it apart as a holy day."*[6]

All God was doing was mandating margin in people's lives. He tells us, "I know you have the ability to work seven days a week. But it's not good for you! I know what your performance ability is, but I also know at how many RPMs your life ought to be running, so I want to mandate margin for you!"

If you begin to read in the Old Testament, you'll find this principle all the way through. Regularly, God said, "I want you to take one year, and I want you to let a field rest. I don't want you to plant anything." Why? Because God was mandating margin. God understands something we have a hard time understanding: *Busy-ness is the enemy of intimacy.* The most powerful man to ever walk on the face of the earth, undeniably, was Jesus. When you study His life in detail and read about the rhythm of His life, you will begin to see that He was a man who understood the principle of margin.

Taking a Sabbath can be hard to justify in our culture, but we need to remember that as believers, we are called to not be of this world. The rhythm of regular rest is good for our souls. The discipline of Sabbath helps us keep margin in our lives.

No margin leads to *fatigue*. Margin brings **energy**.

No margin is *red ink*. Margin is **black ink**.

No margin is *anxiety*. Margin is **security**.

No margin is *culture*. Margin is **counterculture**.

No margin is *the disease* of our time. Margin is **its cure**.

"For of His fullness we have all received, and grace upon grace."[7] God gives us grace on top of grace—like the waves in the ocean coming in an endless rhythm of renewal and refreshing. He has a limitless supply of grace. He encourages us to learn the unforced rhythms of grace, and in so doing, grants us the opportunity to live freely and lightly.

I have found this to be true in my 25-plus year battle with mental illness: my capacity to overcome is directly tied to my consistency in these areas of my life. Let me repeat it. Consistency creates capacity.

Regular confession—coming into agreement with who God is and who He says I am—is an essential rhythm in my life. Personal worship empowers me to overcome the lies that hold me back. Regularly getting my heart rate up strengthens my heart not only physically, but emotionally. If God uses all things for good (and I've staked my life on that fact), then one of the good things that have come out of difficult seasons has been the understanding and practice of this truth.

"He restores my soul."[8]

Jesus did not come merely to save you for a world that is to come. He came to RESTORE you in the world in which you now live. Jesus came to bring restoration to your heart. He came to bring light to the dark places in your soul. He came to heal where you have been wounded because of the reality of living in a fallen world. Jesus wants to walk us through the broken places of our lives and restore our hearts and souls. One of the critical aspects of this journey we are taking together is opportunity. We have an opportunity to begin to walk out this healing with the Lord. It's not going to come in an instantaneous moment—we are not going to microwave this process of restoration and healing. It's going to be a long walk in one direction. I love the words of Max Lucado, "If there are a thousand steps between you and God ... if there are a thousand steps between you and your healing ... God will take nine

> JESUS CAME NOT MERELY TO SAVE YOU FOR A WORLD TO COME, BUT TO RESTORE YOU IN THE WORLD IN WHICH YOU NOW LIVE

hundred and ninety-nine, folks, but you have got to take one. You've got to take one!"

In his book, *Waking the Dead,* John Eldredge writes these words:

> *Everyone carries a wound. I have never met someone without one. No matter how good your life may have seemed to you, you live in a broken world, filled with broken people. Your mother and father, no matter how wonderful, couldn't have been perfect. She is a daughter of Eve, and he is a son of Adam. So, there was no crossing through this country without taking a wound. And every wound, whether it is assaultive or passive, delivers with it, a message. The message feels final and true—true—because it is delivered with such force. Our reaction to it shapes our personality in very significant ways, because from that wound—from that message—flows the false self.*[9]

"Every one of us carries the wounds of misinterpreted messages in the character formation of our lives." Some of us, whether we are 25 or 65, are still battling the demons of those messages we chose to believe from a very early age. We all face these wounds, that is the challenge before every one of us. We are all battling the wrong messages we received in the formative time of our lives. Those messages are giving us not only a false sense of ourselves; they are giving us a false sense of who God is. Jesus came to "heal the brokenhearted and to bind up their wounds,"[10] because God understood that we ALL are going to deal with these wounds in our lives. Consistent practice of the unforced rhythms of grace heals our broken hearts and binds up our wounds.

God wants you to find your identity in Him. He wants you to see yourself as HE sees you. Spend time with Him, spend time in His word. Spend time finding rest and peace in His rhythms of grace. I would like to share this prayer:

Lord, I ask You to bless us in our desire to set regular rhythms of grace. Bless us in our struggle with whatever thorns and limps we have. Pour out Your healing touch on our lives. I pray for the freedom our heart longs for. Father, I speak against the voice of worthlessness and guilt and unworthiness Satan wants to pour on our hearts today. Set us free from the need to be busy. Release us from the idols of packed calendars and long to-do lists.

Lord, give us the power to release control. Teach us how to let go of those things over which we have no control, so they will no longer control us.

Father, I pray You create tremendous testimony from my life—from our lives. In weakness give grace. Allow us to see the real power of Jesus. Give us greater trust and dependence on You than we have ever had before. You promise that out of our struggles, You will bring about good. We thank You for grace and for the freedom You bring each of us.

Thank you, Lord, for coming to set us free.

ENDNOTES

1. Proverbs 12:25.
2. Matthew 11:28-29.
3. Psalm 94:19.
4. 1 Peter 5:7.
5. Exodus 20:8-10a.
6. Exodus 20:10b-11.
7. John 1:16.
8. Psalm 23:1-3.
9. *Waking the Dead* by John Eldredge. © 2003, 2016. Published by Nelson Books. Nashville, Tennessee.
10. Psalm 147:3.

LORD, TEACH US HOW TO
LET GO OF THOSE THINGS
OVER WHICH WE HAVE NO
CONTROL, SO THEY WILL
NO LONGER CONTROL US

CHAPTER SEVEN

BLACK AND WHITE

There are no grey areas. That's the best way to describe the way I was raised to look at life. My family gathered with other believers on Sunday, every Sunday, where we heard preachers regularly use words like "always" and "never."

God **always** does _____.

God **never** does _____.

Black and white.

Monochrome.

I loved this kind of teaching because it fit my personality so well. My whole world revolved around sports back then. Not only did I get black and white preaching on the weekends, my coaches preached a similar black and white gospel as well. If you work harder than the other team you'll always win. Short cuts in training and preparation never work. The fact is, I liked looking at the world through monochrome lenses. It made me feel safe. It made me feel like I knew what to expect. It gave me a sense of control.

My early days of ministry were filled with black and white messages. I first taught messages with absolute language to high school students and then adults. I shared these messages with deep passion and conviction and saw very little wrong with my methodology. Back in those days, I wasn't alone in the comfort zone of always and never. Other pastors and ministers I followed and watched also found security in formulas: A+B=C theology about God brings peace of mind in a world filled with unknowns.

Those lenses got shattered about a year into my battle with panic attacks. Formulas that I had believed and had been teaching to others weren't working for me. I was declaring by faith that I was healed, but the terrifying nights of a racing heart and no sleep were still happening. I confessed and repented of every sin I could think of (and some that I'm sure I made up) but God wasn't fixing my problem. I went through seasons of believing that there was a problem with me—if I just believed more, listened to more worship music, prayed better, or was a better person in general, then God would do something. I also went weeks believing that there must be something wrong with God.

He didn't listen. If He did, I would be cured.

He didn't care. If He did, I would be cured.

Black and white.

I convinced myself that everything He said in the Bible was only true for other people. I felt like a guy with terrible vision who had lost his last pair of glasses. I was flying blind, and I vacillated between anger, bitterness, and a deep sadness.

It was the Apostle Paul's famous words about his thorn in the flesh that started the process of my finding a new pair of lenses to see the world through. Sometimes when you're reading the Bible, you have to see yourself before you can see what God is trying to say to you.

Three times I pleaded with the Lord to take it away from me. But he said to me, "My grace is sufficient for you, for my power is made perfect in weakness."

Therefore, I will boast all the more gladly about my weaknesses, so that Christ's power may rest on me. That is why, for Christ's sake, I delight in weaknesses, in insults, in hardships, in persecutions, in difficulties. For when I am weak, then I am strong.[1]

Paul's story was my story.

Paul had a problem that he called his "thorn in the flesh." Scholars have debated for years on what his problem really was. I think Paul was vague so that all of us could see his pain as our pain. I am convinced that he was having panic attacks. Others believe that it was depression or diabetes or whatever is making them feel less than. All that we know for certain is that whatever was happening, it was painful and debilitating.

You ever had a thorn in your flesh? Check.

Paul prayed at least three times for healing in an area of his life that was so troubling he described it as "a messenger of Satan." Many times in the middle of the night I told Mika I would see red eyes in the corner of our room. I saw the same eyes the first night I started writing this book.

You ever feel demonic presence? Check.

God didn't say yes to Paul's request. He prayed three times asking Him to take it away. Was it a literal count, or just an indicator of asking for it on multiple occasions? I don't know, but I lost count of the number of times I have asked God to heal me and take my anxiety away.

You ever asked, "Please God, take this away"? Check.

It was Paul's response to God's no that blew my mind. I read it over and over again. He wasn't going to hide his pain, he actually used the word "boast." He didn't even say that with God's help he could endure his problem. He used the word "delight." I remember where I was sitting when this truth hit me. You can insert in your mind a picture of a light bulb going off here.

Life is not black and white. God is not monochrome. It is possible to find joy, peace, freedom, and hope in the gray areas of life. God lives in the grey areas. In fact, the only way to find freedom is to shatter your old glasses, to see the world as He sees the world. It's one of the reasons Paul says later that we are transformed by changing the way we think.

THE FIRST STEP TO CHANGING THE WAY YOU THINK IS TO LET GOD CHANGE THE WAY YOU SEE

The first step to changing the way you think is to let God change the way you see. Change happens under tension. Tension brings stress. We often see stress as something to be avoided, but I've found the stress of "both/and" to be more of a freedom giver than my early desires for "either/or." What do I mean? I'm glad you asked.

Does God heal people today?

Absolutely.

I've tried to follow Paul's example and be open about my battle with panic attacks. I've talked about this thorn on television, in my home church, and in churches around the country. At the end of most of these talks, I've prayed for literally thousands of people who are looking for healing in the area of mental health. I've gotten hugs in the room and emails days later where people have shared a supernatural moment of God's healing touch. They usually describe it as a feeling of something being lifted off of them.

That has NEVER been my experience.

Think about it—God uses the prayer of a guy with anxiety to lift anxiety off of someone else and yet doesn't heal the guy. Yes, there are times where I think, "Why not me?" But I've seen that movie before, and I know where that kind of thinking leads.

Does it still suck?

Yep. Does God still use it?

Yes. Does He still heal?

I have witnessed the healings first-hand, so yes He does.

Is it possible that I'm next? For sure, but there are no guarantees. It's a **not yet** kind of experience.

I know God uses my story in the lives of people. The public nature of my job has led to hundreds if not thousands of opportunities through the years to sit across tables from others, especially men, and talk about their struggles with panic and anxiety. Our stories have different layers and details, but the questions, the temptations, and the fears are always the same. It's not what I say that helps them—sometimes I don't say much at all. It's what they see: a fifty-something-year-old guy who loves his family, is grateful for his job, and loves his life. The picture gives them hope.

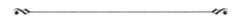

God uses broken people, and I am grateful that He does. I am redeemed, restored, and whole in the eyes of Jesus. And yet, at times I still feel broken and weak. There are seasons when I can't sleep, have a hard time eating, and experience waves of anxiety that inevitably lead into the pit of depression. In those moments, I have never thought to myself, *This is great, I'm going to really help someone with they hear about this.* But it is in those dark places that I feel His power at work. I feel His strength the most when I'm at my weakest. I love being used by God. Panic attacks suck the life out of me. God breathes life back into me. "The Lord is near to the brokenhearted."[2] I love the near part, but the brokenhearted part is not at the top of my list.

It's in the tension of this *not yet* reality that my faith gets tested and ultimately grows. I don't have to like it to know it's true. Real life is found in relationship with God. That relationship is **initiated** by God through the sacrificial love of His Son, Jesus Christ. "While I was still sinning," Jesus chose to initiate a relationship by dying on the cross for me.[3] He moved towards me long before I even looked His way. Why? Because his relationship with me is unconditional. Healthy relationships work that way. A conditional relationship is no real relationship at all. It is in this where I have found freedom.

I spent so much of my life putting conditions on my relationship with God. Can you relate to putting conditions on God even though He loves you unconditionally? God was Monty Hall and my life was *Let's Make A Deal.* I needed Him to do something, fix something, right all of the wrongs in my world—*then* I would be okay, *then* WE would be okay. It was black and white thinking. But God lives in the gray.

It's not either/or.

It's both/and.

There's a beauty in the tension of weak and strong, pain and nearness, sadness and joy. I would love a miracle. I don't need one to love Jesus. I don't need one to believe that He's with me.

When we read the story of the prodigal son, we focus most of our attention on him. But let's look at his older brother:

> *Meanwhile, the older son was in the field. When he came near the house, he heard music and dancing. So, he called one of the servants and asked him what was going on. "Your brother has come," he replied, "and your father has killed the fattened calf because he has him back safe and sound."*
>
> *The older brother became angry and refused to go in. So, his father went out and pleaded with him. But he answered his father, "Look! All these years I've been slaving for you and never disobeyed your orders. Yet you never gave me even a young goat so I could celebrate with my friends. But when this son of yours who has squandered your property with prostitutes comes home, you kill the fattened calf for him!"*[4]

The older brother was a black and white kind of guy. His little brother had wasted his inheritance. He should be punished. Bad people get bad things. He had stayed and worked with his father and picked up the slack of his brother's mistakes. He should be rewarded. Garth Brooks should show up and sing. Pappas Bros should cater an all you can eat meat fest. Good people should get good things. But the father in this story didn't wear black and white glasses. He was so filled with joy that his rebellious, irresponsible, broken son came home that he threw the biggest bash his little corner had ever seen. Food and laughter and music. It was epic.

And the son looking through life with his black and white lens missed the party.

I spent way too many years living like that older brother. I missed too much joy that my Father wanted to give me. That's not what I want any more. I don't want to miss the heart of my Father. I don't want to look back at my life and say, "Wow, I missed a great party." I don't have to have all the answers, I just want to know my Father. For me, that's what freedom looks like.

> I DON'T HAVE TO HAVE ALL THE ANSWERS, I JUST WANT TO KNOW MY FATHER

Shatter your old glasses.

Be transformed by His love.

Leave black and white behind.

Embrace the grey.

Know your Father.

ENDNOTES

1. 2 Corinthians 12:8-10.
2. Psalm 34:18.
3. Romans 5:8.
4. Luke 15:25-30.

IT'S IN THE TENSION OF
OUR "NOT YET" REALITY
THAT OUR FAITH
GETS TESTED AND
ULTIMATELY GROWS

CHAPTER EIGHT

BE A GOBY

We are all familiar with the epic picture of salmon swimming upstream in the Pacific Northwest. Great salmon runs are where thousands of fish swim upstream to spawn and then die. It doesn't end well for them. I've listened to hundreds of motivational speeches about salmon. Salmon have been a perfect message illustration to show me how I have to fight for my purpose and how important it is for me to develop a spirit of endurance.

I love the imagery of salmon but let me tell you what I like more; the goby fish—*Sicyopterus stimpsoni*. Also known as the "inching climber," few people have ever even heard about the humble goby. These fish leave the saltwater sanctuary where they were carried downstream and deposited as baby fish and in their adolescence, they re-enter the fresh-water rivers surrounding the Hawaiian Islands. Like salmon, goby fish also swim upstream and overcome great obstacles in order to spawn. But in my humble opinion, the goby has the salmon beat. Not only do they swim tirelessly against the raging current as they migrate, they must also scale rocks behind great waterfalls using two tiny suction cups on their body and push upward with their fins as they scale upwards inch-by-painstaking-inch to reach a safe haven.

The goby is a small fish, only a few inches long. If you caught one, you would probably throw it back. So, their daring climb up a 350-foot rock face is comparable to you or me scaling Mount Everest three times![1]

I like the goby for a couple of reasons: partly because they don't just go up there, have eggs, and die. They live on for years, playing in the river rapids they worked so hard to reach. I like the goby more than salmon mostly because of what happens to them when they begin to climb. The fight to swim upstream radically changes this little fish. The goby is transformed in the battle to swim upstream.

David wrote that "the heavens declare the glory of God."[2] He wasn't saying that the majesty of God is seen only in a sunrise or mountain view. David was explaining that we best see God's **intent** in His creation. You want to know what God is up to when you find yourself in turbulent waters? Look at the goby. Let's talk about turbulence for a moment.

WE'LL NEVER BE ENTIRELY FREE UNTIL WE GET A GOD-SIZED PICTURE OF WHAT WALKING IN FREEDOM MEANS

I think walking in freedom for you and me is not obtained in the still waters. We'll never be entirely free until we get a God-sized picture of what walking in freedom means. Freedom is when depression, disappointment, or disillusionment take you downstream, but you fight. Freedom is when you use the little bit of strength you have, and even the strength you don't have, and you fight your way upstream: inch-by-painstaking-inch. Sometimes your head goes underwater for a moment. Most of the time, you're not sure you're going to make it. But you refuse to go with the flow. You fight to swim upstream. You fight to reach the waters of your origin—the place from which you were created to dwell before you were swept downstream in the raging current of life.

Freedom is not about the absence of something.

Freedom is about the presence of Someone.

We all experience pain. In some seasons, it may feel like we can't keep the pain from coming. We tend to spend our time asking God "why" questions and begging Him to take away the ache. Maybe you find yourself in a difficult season right now. The challenge of the difficult seasons and the pain those seasons bring is to allow that pain to take you to places you never wanted to go.

Turbulent waters.

Swimming upstream.

Fighting gravity's pull.

Dreams of still waters dominate our depressing days and our anxious nights. We need to understand that this mythical moment when we're not going to struggle, when it's not going to be hard, when there's not going to be turbulent waters is *never going to come*. That moment is never going to come. The call of God in our lives is freedom. Freedom is not the absence of those turbulent waters. Freedom is the supernatural Spirit-given power to keep swimming upstream.

The goby fish shows me God's ultimate purpose is to change me. The difference between me and a goby? I get to decide. It's my choice whether I get bitter or get better. I don't get to choose the water, but I do get to determine what I will look like on the other side of the rapids. God is using these moments for my good. He is trying to build my character and change my perspective. He is positioning me for maximum impact in the lives of those around me. I can cross my arms and bow my neck and blame Him for not fixing my problems or I can begin to allow him to shape me into His best version of the man He created me to be. I want to be a goby.

We all have our battles—our limp, our thorns. Your battle may be panic and anxiety, like mine. But your struggle may be different. A battle is anything that causes us to feel less than. Your marriage blows up. Your kid rebels. The bills are piled too high. Your health is challenged. For me, it's panic attacks that come at the stupidest times for no reason.

When I'm feeling "less than," the things that begin to present in my life are, number one, I have a hard time eating; number two, I have a hard time sleeping; and number three, it causes me to want to isolate. Now, you may be at the other end of the spectrum. When hard times come, you may want to eat everything in sight. You may want to medicate. Guess what the result is of me not eating, not sleeping, and isolating? Anybody got an idea? I go farther down in the ditch. And guess what? I have more panic and anxiety—not less. I see myself as defeated, so I yield to things which defeat me until I fulfill my own prophecy.

I have noticed that when I find myself in those seasons, it's incredibly important for me to do the very things I do not want to do so that I did not become a self-fulfilling prophecy. I think that freedom is growing in the ability to swim upstream. As a leader, as a person to whom God has given influence, the rhythm of your life must be to swim upstream. Swim upstream even when the water is turbulent.

Spiritual disciplines are imperative to prepare you for tempestuous moments that are coming your way. We need to see the Spirit-given determination to keep swimming when life doesn't go our way. I want to live in a rhythm of life where I'm doing things that I'm not naturally inclined to do, but I know are good for me because they give me life. Do you know what those things are for you? I'm not talking about happy things, just the things you enjoy. I'm talking about things that might be hard, but fortify your spirit, strengthen your mind, nourish your soul, and prepare you for the battles that are already coming your way.

- Do you know what those things are in your life?

- What disciplines do you need to cultivate to keep you in a place of readiness?

One of mine is exercise. I hate exercise. The only runner's high I get is when I quit. My decision to make my heart beat fast and exercise is because it helps me swim upstream. I have found it is imperative for me; it's a non-negotiable for me in battling this thing that makes me feel less than. Do you know when it's the toughest for me to do? It's hardest when I'm in the middle of a season of those attacks. Because my heart is already beating fast with panic, so I get on the elliptical, and I'm on about two minutes and guess what happens? My heart starts beating fast. I go, "Oh crap, here we go again!" and I want to quit—and that's the moment I need it the most. Causing my heart to beat fast with exercise cancels the power anxiety exerts to make it beat fast with panic. One is healthy, within my influence; the other destructive, beyond my control.

What is it that you need the most? What price are you willing to pay to find the life you've always been looking for? Freedom isn't the absence of turbulent water. It is the ability to swim upstream when life is trying to take you out. But you have to set yourself up to be successful. You have to grow the muscles you will need to swim upstream.

Some things set you up for failure. These are things that aren't necessarily bad, but they are not good for *you* because of *your* unique battle. I mentioned before that for me, one thing is scary movies. I don't go to scary movies. You may like scary movies like *Poltergeist* or something, but I'm going next door to watch a Disney movie. I have an anxiety disorder.

My dad is 85 now and has a lot of time on his hands. I think he watches the news five times a day. He's into all these police shows, too. He always wants to talk to me about what he saw on the news or the latest episode of COPS. I finally had to tell him that I don't watch those shows. Why? The content of those shows makes me feel tense! If the genre on the DVR says suspense or horror, I'm out. I know those things don't put me in a position where I can swim upstream because of the challenges I have in this life.

- Do you know what those things are in your life?
- What things do you need to stay away from?

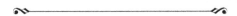

I like the goby fish because two days into the climb up the waterfall, its body physically changes. Its mouth gets longer. Its jaw drops. Why? So, it'll have enough suction to grab onto a rock and climb up a waterfall, and so that it can eat differently. Even their diet changes!

To survive the climb, the goby needs to eat the algae off the rocks that will give it the strength to get to its destination.[3]

The transformation we all want comes in the upstream rowing that we all must do. It's the picture Paul talks about for anyone that's behind; it's straining toward what is ahead. The physical, emotional, and especially the physical condition you want, gets built, not when it's easy, but when you push through the hard times. Repeated resistance is what builds muscle. It's in the struggle that you are changed. God transforms you, and He transforms you by better positioning you to win whatever battle that's in front of you.

> IT'S IN THE MIDDLE OF THE STRUGGLE WHERE WE ARE CHANGED

You can be like my one friend and spend all your time asking yourself:

- Why is this happening to me?
- Why is my marriage blowing up?
- Why do my kids rebel?
- Why do I have depression?
- Why am I battling anxiety attacks?

Or you can put your trust in God, put your head down, and swim.

The person I want to be is not going to be found because I never have another panic attack. The person I want to be is going to be found because I find strength to endure in the middle of those attacks. There's not a day goes by I don't ask God to take them away from me. I have no doubt it is within God's ability, and it is God's heart for me to be free from those things. But until he does, in these "not yet" moments, there is tremendous work He does in my life.

The older I've gotten, the more I think about the end of my days. I think about the end of my days on earth. Not in a morbid way but in a much more reflective way. I know the younger you are, the weirder that seems. I want people who are close to me—the ones who are paying attention—to say I fought the good fight. I finished the race. I want to finish well.

For a long time, I lived in a place where I asked God to fix what was broken in me. I've wanted Him to snap His fingers and take my thorn from me. Now, I ask Him to refine me as I swim upstream. I ask Him to help me swim well. I make an effort every day to do the things that bring me life. I choose things that restore my soul. I avoid like the plague the things that keep me from the life I want.

People need to see you swim upstream well. The world needs to see the community of believers swimming upstream well. That's where you will find a life filled with freedom.

Do hard things.

Play scared.

Do the things that make your knees knock a little bit.

Be a goby.

> Though He slay me, yet will I hope in Him; I will surely defend my ways to His face. Indeed, this will turn out for my deliverance ...[4] God's now at my side and I'm not afraid; who would dare lay a hand on me? [5]

ENDNOTES

1. *Waterfall-climbing Fish Performs Evolutionary Feat.* © 2014 National Science Foundation. Posted 03 February, 2014 by Miles O'Brien, Science Nation Correspondent, and Marsha Watton, Science Nation Producer. Retrieved 13 November, 2019 from: https://scienceblog. com/70216/waterfall-climbing-fish-performs-evolutionary-feat/.

2. Psalm 19:1.

3. *Determined Fish Climb Waterfalls with Special Sucker Mouths* © 2013 Smithsonian.com. Posted 07 January, 2013 by Rachel Nower. Retrieved 13 November, 2019 from: https://www.smithsonianmag.com/science-nature/ determined-fish-climb-waterfalls-with-special-sucker-mouths-393459/.

4. Job 13:15-16a.

5. Psalm 118:6, MSG.

FREDOM ISN'T
THE ABSENCE OF
TURBULENT WATER,
IT IS THE ABILITY TO
SWIM UPSTREAM
WHEN LIFE IS TRYING
TO TAKE YOU OUT

CHAPTER NINE

EVEN IN THE NOT YET

We drove north out of Denton in complete silence. Tears began to well up in both of our eyes. It was too painful to address each other, so we both stared straight ahead. Neither of us wanted to look at the other, knowing if our eyes met, it would just make things worse. This wasn't the first time we had said goodbye to our kids. It wasn't the first time we had kissed our two grandsons and driven away, but no matter how many times we did it, it never seemed to get any easier. There was no amount of emotional preparation that made parting company any less painful. Each time we said goodbye, it took the wind right out of our spirits. Nothing about the endings of our visits was happy. Finally, I dared to look at Mika. Her eyes caught mine in a knowing gaze, she sighed and said, "I just never thought we'd find ourselves here—I miss those boys already."

I nodded in agreement. For some crazy reason, we had assumed that we would always have a front-row seat during all our grandkids' growing up years. I had a plan in my head that we would have little ones around us all the time. I didn't have to worry about what I would miss because I believed they would be living their lives right around the corner. Seeing them load up for the drive home to Mississippi was a reminder that God often has a different plan for our lives. Most times, His plans are much different than we had ever imagined. Visits were always great—but still way too short, and not nearly as often as any of us would like. Here's the thing, everything about their life in is excellent. Grant, my son-in-law, has a great job, they are part of a life-giving church, and they share real community with good friends. It was just that all these blessings, in the opinion of Papa T and Honey, are taking place for them in the wrong state. The truth is, our daughter and her family are happy. It's just not what I had planned.

I concentrated on the road ahead, pushing back emotion the best I could. I wrestled with what was bad and ugly about this situation and ended up finding some good in it after all. A few more moments of silence passed between us before I said, "Mika, isn't it crazy, though, how God has filled in the gaps for us?" My mind flooded with the faces of all the spiritual sons and daughters we have had the privilege of investing in. One of the blessings that Mika and I are so thankful for is the relationships we have built over decades while serving at Cross Timbers. Pouring into the next generation of leaders is a shared passion for Mika and me. We count it a high honor to be able to pray for and walk alongside the mothers and fathers raising their little ones all around us. I started talking about the two young ones down the street who God had divinely placed in our lives just as our kids made their move eight hours away. We got to be surrogate grandparents for a season. I smiled in spite of myself, impossible not to as I counted these blessings. Mika nodded her head, remembering with me as I talked. We were able to find joy and happiness even in this bittersweet space. Then we both went silent again. We've been married for over thirty years and have gotten really good at knowing what the other is thinking without either of us having to say a word.

We are usually on the same page, and I knew we were both grateful for the blessings, and finally, I said out loud, "But, it's not what we want." Mika shook her head in agreement, fresh tears surfaced, and she said, "I just never thought I'd find myself here."

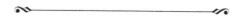

I never dreamed in my twenties than in my fifties I would be writing a book about a twenty-five-year battle with anxiety and panic. In fact, ten years into this journey, I remember telling Mika that one day I'd be writing a book about the complete healing God gave me from this emotional illness. I have been waiting to write it until I could testify to the healing, totally free from anxiety. But here I am, still battling panic, questioning if I am qualified to write about it even without the "victory." I meet so many who, like me, find themselves in a place they never dreamed they would be. If you've made it this far in this book, you probably have said words like, "I just never thought I'd find myself divorced ... or addicted ... or broke ... or grieving ... or _____." Life hasn't gone or isn't going, the way you dreamed it would.

You are wounded and weary. You are disappointed and a little ticked off about where you find yourself.

The writer of Hebrews points out that there learned obedience in suffering. "Son though he was, he learned obedience from what he suffered."[1] It is impossible to grow in faith unless we have something to overcome. Your faith is often built from your problems. We can learn from our suffering.

Keep in mind, problems do not always symbolize the absence of God in your life. We all want to stand up and sing *Oceans* by Hillsong, but we don't want to get into the water up to our necks! In your journey and in my journey, we must continually remind ourselves that there are opportunities in challenges. Our perspective in problems is where the enemy fights us. What makes us different is that God is at work to form and shape us in His image through our problems. We have to reframe our thinking—shift our perspective so that we see the hard spaces as a place where God is actively shaping us into His image. Because of Him, we can have courage amid our problems. Too often we try to make things just right so we can finally be happy. Give up the need to be happy and let God teach you something in the tension.

Let's think about it this way: sometimes problems are just problems. Sometimes towers fall. It's not your fault all the time, and then sometimes it is. Let's own our individual responses in each of our situations and seasons no matter who's fault it is. Let's take ownership of how we respond. It takes courage to own your own crap and be satisfied regardless of your circumstances. It takes courage to be authentically positive in the midst of your problems. There is no life in complaining. Let's live—give grace and stand together in love. I know this is a radical way to live in this space and time, but it is a better way to exist. Pray that God will give you the courage to own what you need to own. Ask for forgiveness, and in that, you will find so much more than happiness. Christ in you is the hope of glory, and in that truth, you can find real joy.

You must step toward freedom. Now that you see your struggle for what it is and you are ready for God to do something, begin to walk toward your freedom. Chances are, it took you a long time to walk into your struggle, and it is going to take a while to step out of it. God will probably not hit you with a lightning bolt to fix all your problems. Instead, He will take your hand and walk you down a path that will totally transform you. He will get down to the "why" of your struggle and heal the wounds in your heart.

Your part in the process is to take a step in that direction. Refuse to wallow in your circumstances. Cooperate with God and move with Him. I promise, if you take one step, He will meet you by taking the other ninety-nine.

Taking a step will look different for each person. It may mean joining a group of like-minded people who are also stepping toward freedom. It may mean going to a Christian counselor who can help you gain biblical perspective and submit to God's path for your life. There are Christian counseling centers all over the country. There are loving people in your community, waiting to connect meaningfully with you. You weren't designed to heal on your own, don't try.

For some of you, stepping toward healing is a maintenance issue. Maybe you've been through counseling, and you have the tools you need to walk in freedom, you just have to do it. We must never grow weary of walking out our healing. Satan only needs the slightest opportunity to bring us back to bondage.

I love how Paul puts it to his spiritual son Timothy, "Spend your time and energy in training yourself for spiritual fitness."[2]

Take the time and trouble. If you want to be free, you must begin to walk in the direction of freedom.

Friend, this is the beginning of a great journey for you. God wants you to discover the peace of living in beautiful communion with Him. It won't always be comfortable, and all your problems are not going to disappear.

> IF YOU WANT TO BE FREE, YOU MUST BEGIN TO WALK IN THE DIRECTION OF FREEDOM

The goal is not a problem-free life; instead, it is abundant life. Run home to Him. He is waiting to throw a party, to cover you with His robe of righteousness, to give you the shoes of the Son and the ring of His glory. Allow Him to walk you down a path of healing that will not only set you free but will also set your children free.

I have been sharing my story with you in these pages so you could see that I've been where you are. I may not know the minute details of your stories or the debilitating places you have found yourself in. But I am not just saying I understand how you feel; I actually know how you feel. The fight not to feel "less than" is a familiar battle for me. If I had the privilege to sit down with you over a cup of coffee and you told me your story, I would want you to walk away knowing these three things:

1. GOD ALWAYS PROVIDES

> *But seek his kingdom, and these things will be given to you*
> *as well. Do not be afraid, little flock, for your Father has*
> *been pleased to give you the kingdom.*[3]

God always provides—He just doesn't always provide what I want. If I have learned anything through this season, it's that the battle for my heart is ultimately about embracing the imperfect. It's a painfully sanctifying thing to begin to accept and even find gratitude in God's gifts on His terms and in His timing. What I desire is to never wake up with my heart racing and my chest pounding. He's given me is the grace to be "hard-pressed but not crushed" in those moments when it feels like my world is spinning out of control. Is it what I want? No! I pray for supernatural healing from panic and anxiety every day. But I don't need the miracle of healing to be free. God's promises are not about delivering me *from* something, He promises to deliver me *through* something. The provision He provides may not always look like complete healing. The spiritual truth in that is that He is still there, He is still providing even if I don't experience complete healing. It is the mystery of His provision. God always provides, it just may not always look like what we want or what we thought.

I hate panic attacks, but I can say with all honesty that I've sensed God's power and presence in those moments, unlike any other times in my life. I have decided to be grateful for what He's given me, even if it's not what I ask Him for the most. I joke with my son telling him that being a grandfather is about giving my grandkids what they want—it is his job as a father to provide them with what they need. I think I'm finally learning that God is a Father, not a Grandfather. I'm finding peace in that reality.

2. GOD IS AT WORK

For it is God who works in you to will and to act in order to fulfill his good purpose.[4]

God is at work even when it feels like He is not. There have been many times through the years that I have raised my fist and shouted at God, "Where are you? Why won't you fix this? What is wrong with me? What is wrong with you?" I never saw it in the moment, but I can say now with full confidence that He was at work, always. He has taught me how to minister out of my brokenness and weakness rather than only through my strengths. I feel released from the need to have all the answers for you or for me. Trust me, that's Him at work! He's built compassion into my heart and spirit for people who are hurting. He has given me an awareness that I'm convinced would have never come without this battle. Most of all, He has been working to teach me how to trust Him, not to sing a song about trusting, but to really trust Him—to trust that He's got me and the things I love the most under control.

I've discovered that I want to be an overcomer, I just don't like having things to overcome. *Oceans (Where Feet May Fail)* is an excellent song to sing in church, I just don't actually want to feel like I'm drowning in "deepest waters" when "oceans rise." I don't know what it is that you are facing, but panic attacks make me feel like I'm doing precisely that—drowning. In those moments, all I have is Jesus. If He doesn't get me through, I'm done. It's an ugly, hard, crappy, and beautiful place to be. He's changing me, even though He's not fixing me. He is teaching me that He is at work, even when it feels like He's not there.

3. GOD'S PEACE IS POSSIBLE WITHOUT PERFECTION

You will keep in perfect peace those whose minds are steadfast, because they trust in you.[5]

I have this memory of sitting in class as a third grader beginning to panic as the teacher passed out our graded math tests. I wasn't scared of failing, I was anxiety-ridden about not making a 100. As crazy as it may sound, that moment clearly defines one of (if not the biggest) problems in my life: the need to be perfect—in school, in church, in relationships, in life. I lived many years under the false and debilitating belief that happiness could only be found in perfection. The problem was (and is) that perfection on this planet is impossible. My marriage, my friendships, my job performance, my parenting, my walk with Jesus are all imperfect. That's why I believed that if I was fully known, I couldn't be fully loved because only perfect people were loved perfectly. That's why I told my first counselor that anything less than having no panic attacks was unacceptable. For God to be real and for me to be whole, I had to be perfect in the anxiety department.

I have since learned how toxic that kind of thinking can be to a man's soul, and how contrary that thought is to the heart of God. I haven't stopped believing that God can heal me, but my wounds don't define me. Scars can be a beautiful thing—they bring hope to bleeding and bruised people that God loves wholeheartedly and accepts unconditionally no matter how "imperfect" we may feel. So, since that first day in my counselor's office, my goals have changed. If the Lord's answer to my most often spoken prayer continues to be "No," and if I fight panic until my last day on earth, I can say with all my heart that it is well with my soul. I can truthfully testify that God is still providing and working, He is still giving me peace in the midst of all the mess. He is perfect in the middle of all my imperfection.

Most of us are living in the ***not yet***. If that is where you find yourself today, then the greatest decision of your life at this moment would be to ignore the voices which keep telling you that you're less than because of your challenge. Invite the Christ who lives in you right into the middle of your battle with you. I may not know your situation, but I do know this: God isn't done with you. He's a good Father who gives His kids precisely what they need. He will restore you. Restoration may not look like Him giving you back exactly what it is you've lost, but He will give you the life you've never expected if you'll just keep walking. I'll believe for you

INVITE THE CHRIST WHO LIVES IN YOU RIGHT INTO THE MIDDLE OF YOUR BATTLE WITH YOU when it's hard for you to believe for yourself. You remind me when the pain makes it hard for me to remember the words I've written. Together we can know this—peace is possible, Jesus is real, and your best days are yet ahead.

It takes courage to keep going. It takes courage not to quit. There is power in endurance and in perseverance. The enemy comes at it fully because there is such a blessing on the other side of it. When the problems arise, the way you win, the way I win, is to outlast. We need to outlast our critics.

True confession: The impetus for writing *Not Yet* was emotional health. When I first considered writing these chapters and planning the correlating message series, I was thinking of my battles through the years with panic and anxiety. I was reading article after article about the alarmingly high number of Americans dealing with depression, anxiety, and other emotional challenges. Most of the things I have read are helpful, but for me, incomplete.

In the dark times of my anxiety, I tried a myriad of exercises and techniques to bring me back to some sense of emotional well-being. Knowing that my physical health plays a vital role, I do my best to exercise regularly and be somewhat disciplined about nutrition. I have been intentional about cultivating certain level 10 relationships. These relationships allow me to be completely open and honest about my doubts and struggles during the dark times of my soul. Prolific authors have taught me the value of soul care, and I try, whenever possible, to live a sustainable pace of life. I believe this entire process factors in my emotional health. This work of the soul positions me for true wellness. Even still, on their own, they are not enough.

Through the years, my definition of emotional health has changed.

In my twenties and early thirties, I thought emotional health was the absence of emotional challenges. I bought into religion's lie that if I just prayed enough, studied enough, and did all the right things, God would keep emotional challenges out of my life. That did not work. I got over my religious arrogance about medications to treat the symptoms of these problems and medications helped for a season.

In my mid-thirties and forties, I discovered the concepts of heart wounds and spiritual warfare. I did the excruciatingly difficult work with Christian counselors and faced my wounds, did some major forgiving, and began to understand how my enemy tried to leverage old thought patterns to take me to unhealthy places. Anxiety still reared its ugly head occasionally, leaving me with self-doubt and questioning the work of God in my life.

I started changing when the target changed. It was a seismic shift for me. Not everyone understands it. Many of my charismatic friends think that I've given up on the notion of complete healing. I can assure you that I have not. Others continue to give me articles on nutrition, theology, meditation exercises, and countless other tools to rid me of any panic attacks once and for all. I know they love me and want to see me emotionally healthy. I want that too. But I'm aiming my arrow at a new bull's eye.

I know this will challenge some of you, but I have come to the place where emotional health for me is not the absence of emotional challenges—the absence of anxiety and the tendency towards depression in its aftermath. For me, emotional health is the development of an overcoming spirit.

When anxiety strikes me from time to time, it is the way I respond which indicates my emotional health. Paul talks about "being persecuted but not abandoned, struck down but not destroyed."[6] To me, that is the very definition of an overcoming spirit. It is in the dark moments that God deepens my prayer life and builds my dependence on Him. I am never more relationally healthy than those tough seasons where I learn how to be completely transparent with those closest to me. I don't like the dark nights of the soul seasons that come, but I am learning to appreciate the mighty work that God does in me during them. Sharing my struggles as a pastor discourages the work of the enemy and leverages my weakness for Christ's strength.

It is the work of the Holy Spirit.

He brings wholeness and health and wellness to my soul. He will take weakness and pain and turn them into strength and victory to accomplish His work in my life. Self-help doesn't work. Christ's help is what I'm looking for. That doesn't mean I don't join Him in the process. I am committed to the practice and principles of wellness in the various areas of my life. It's His work that joins with my choices that brings me to a place of an overcoming spirit. The results are joy and peace and hope in a life that brings Him glory.

Keep standing when everything is falling down around you.

Keep walking.

Keep believing.

Keep trusting.

It is well—even in the not yet.

"... and if not, He is still good." [7]

ENDNOTES

1. Hebrews 5:8.
2. 1 Timothy 4:7.
3. Luke 12:30-32.
4. Philippians 2:13.
5. Isaiah 26:3.
6. 2 Corinthians 4:9.
7. See Daniel 3:1-24.

EMOTIONAL HEALTH
IS THE DEVELOPMENT
OF AN OVERCOMING
SPIRIT AS I ALLOW THE
HOLY SPIRIT TO BRING
WHOLENESS, HEALTH, AND
WELLNESS TO MY SOUL

FROM TOBY'S SON

AFTERWORD

This *Not Yet* journey is searching for the answers. It is looking for the black and white and finding only more grey. It is experiencing joy in the midst of great pain. It is living in the in-between. It is seeing the beauty among the brokenness. It is being confused or angry at yourself, at the world, or at God and still being able to trust in His goodness. What's powerful about this *Not Yet* journey is that it isn't a Toby Slough story—it's a human story. Humanity is comprised of *Not Yet* people.

So, just like you have been on a journey through these pages and chapters, I have lived and witnessed the sometimes painful and other times joy-filled moments. I can honestly say that although the road hasn't been without bumps and bruises, I'm truly grateful for what the *Not Yet* has taught me.

I'm grateful that I have seen a picture of what it looks like to be brutally honest even when feeling great shame.

I'm relieved that I have don't have it all figured out to believe. I'm appreciative that I don't have to have it all right to follow God.

I'm amazed that I've seen a glimpse of fullness of God's grace.

I'm grateful that my dad taught me that being a man doesn't mean you always have to "grit your teeth and bear it." He modeled for me that being a man is just as much not being afraid to ask for help when you need it. He demonstrated that being a husband doesn't always mean being the strong leader who doesn't struggle, and loving your wife "as Christ loved the church" means being honest with her—even when it might seem like you look weak.

I'm overcome that even though I will walk through valleys, I can still believe God is with me. I can trust Romans 8—truly NOTHING can separate me from the love of God. I'm not defined by my valley, my challenge, or circumstance. Being in a valley doesn't change my standing with God.

I'm grateful that I have seen in my dad's life a perseverance, an unshakable hope, and a holding on no matter what. Because of that, I'm inspired to live open-hearted, ready to take on the mountain.

God will continue to use the brutal and beautiful *Not Yet* in my life and yours. My hope and prayer is that we can see the divine even in the darkness. And as we journey on, a profound gratefulness will be cultivated deep in our soul that allows us to see all of life as a gift.

—*Ross Slough*

APPENDIX A

NOT YET RESOURCES

Your journey is your journey. I don't know what will help you strengthen your mind and quiet your spirit, but I wanted to put together a list of some things which have really helped me or have allowed me to help others. I hope they will help you too.

— *Toby*

BOOKS

- *Ordering Your Private World* by Gordon MacDonald
- *Rebuilding Your Broken World* by Gordon MacDonald
- *Soul Keeping* by John Ortberg
- *The Life You've Always Wanted* by John Ortberg
- *Fathered by God* by John Eldredge
- *Wild at Heart* by John Eldredge
- *Captivating* by John & Stasi Eldredge
- *In A Pit With A Lion On A Snowy Day* by Mark Batterson
- *For Men Only* by Shaunti & Jeff Feldhahn

- *For Women Only* by Shaunti & Jeff Feldhahn
- *How to Talk So Kids Will Listen & Listen So Kids Will Talk* by Adele Faber & Elaine Mazlish
- *The Connected Child* by Karen B. Purvis, David R. Cross, Wendy Lyons Sunshine
- *Boundaries* by Dr. Henry Cloud & Dr. John Townsend
- *Changes That Heal* by Dr. Henry Cloud
- *Safe People* by Dr. Henry Cloud & Dr. John Townsend
- *Coping with Depression* Siang-Yang Tan, John Ortberg, Jr.
- *Experiencing Grief* by H. Norman Wright
- *The Smart Stepfamily* by Ron Deal
- *Falling Upward* by Richard Rohr

THE 40 I AM^S
(From Chapter 6)

1. A child of God. *Romans 8:16*
2. Redeemed from the hand of the enemy. *Psalms 107:2*
3. Forgiven. *Colossians 1:13-14*
4. Saved by grace through faith. *Ephesians 2:8*
5. Justified. *Romans 5:1*
6. Sanctified. *1 Corinthians 1:2*
7. A new creature. *2 Corinthians 5:17*
8. Partaker of His divine nature. *2 Peter 1:4*
9. Redeemed from the curse of the law. *Galatians 3:13*

10. Delivered from the powers of darkness. *Colossians 1:13*

11. Led by the Spirit of God. *Romans 8:14*

12. A son of God. *Romans 8:14*

13. Kept in safety wherever I go. *Psalms 91:11*

14. Getting all my needs met by Jesus. *Philippians 4:19*

15. Casting all my cares on Jesus. *1 Peter 5:7*

16. Strong in the Lord and in the power of His might. *Ephesians 6:10*

17. Doing all things through Christ who strengthens me. *Philippians 4:13*

18. An heir of God and a joint heir with Jesus. *Romans 8:17*

19. An heir to the blessing of Abraham. *Galatians 3:13-14*

20. Observing and doing the Lord's Commandments. *Deuteronomy 28:12*

21. Blessed coming in and blessed going out. *Deuteronomy 28:6*

22. An heir of eternal life. *1 John 5:11-12*

23. Blessed with all spiritual blessings. *Ephesians 1:3*

24. Healed by His stripes. *1 Peter 2:24*

25. Exercising my authority over the enemy. *Luke 10:19*

26. Above only and not beneath. *Deuteronomy 28:13*

27. More than a conqueror. *Romans 8:37*

28. Establishing God's Word here on earth. *Matthew 16:19*

29. An overcomer by the blood of the Lamb and the word of my testimony. *Revelation 12:11*

30. Daily overcoming the devil. *1 John 4:4*

31. Not moved by what I see. *2 Corinthians 4:18*

32. Walking by faith and not by sight. *2 Corinthians 5:7*

33. Casting down vain imaginations. *2 Corinthians 10:4-5*

34. Bringing every thought into captivity. *2 Corinthians 10:5*

35. Being transformed by renewing my mind. *Romans 12:1-2*

36. A laborer together with God. *1 Corinthians 3:9*

37. The righteousness of God in Christ. *2 Corinthians 5:21*

38. An imitator of Jesus. *Ephesians 5:1*

39. The light of the world. *Matthew 5:14*

40. Blessing the Lord at all times and continually praising Him with my mouth. *Psalms 34:1*

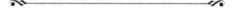

ENCOURAGEMENT

Daily Promise

- www.365promises.com

Father's Love Letter

- www.fathersloveletter.com

Freedom in Christ

- www.ficm.org

SUPPORT

Celebrate Recovery

- www.celebraterecovery.com

Divorce Care

- www.divorcecare.org

Grief Share

- www.griefshare.org

Family Grace

- https://mentalhealthgracealliance.org

Mending The Soul

- https://mendingthesoul.org/

ONLINE RESOURCES:

People of the Second Chance

- www.secondchance.org

Better Help

- www.betterhelp.com

MentalHealth.gov

- www.mentalhealth.gov

Child Mind Institute

- www.childmind.org

National Institute of Mental Health

- *Panic Disorder: When Fear Overwhelms*—https://www.nimh.nih.gov/health/publications/panic-disorder-when-fear-overwhelms/index.shtml

American Psychological Association

- *Answers to Your Questions about Panic Disorder*—https://www.apa.org/topics/anxiety/panic-disorder

Center for Clinical Interventions

- *Panic Stations: Coping with Panic Attacks*—https://www.cci.health.wa.gov.au/resources/looking-after-yourself/panic

APPENDIX B

MEET THE AUTHOR

After graduating from Abilene Christian University in 1986, Toby Slough began his ministry career working with high school students in San Antonio, Texas. During these years, he traveled around the country speaking to teens and youth workers.

Toby and his family moved to Southlake, Texas in 1993 when he became the Preaching Minister for the Southlake Boulevard Church. Here God began to birth in him a dream to plant a church for hurting and broken people in the rural area of Argyle, Texas.

In 2000, Toby, Mika, and twelve families began Cross Timbers Church in the back of a bar. God blessed these humble beginnings and has been building, shaping, and refining the cornerstone foundations at Cross Timbers ever since. God expresses His amazing, abundant work through the multiple ministry streams that make up the Cross Timbers community. There are two vibrant, thriving campuses in North Texas and we are developing a community center model to meet the changing dynamics of local needs. God has gone before us every step of the way as we carry out the vision of loving God and loving people, passionate to develop and send 10,000 Difference Makers into our communities locally and around the world.

Toby and Mika have been married for over thirty-four years. (He married way over his head!) Together they have two children and five grandchildren:

- Bailey (daughter) and Grant have three children—Gideon, Micah, and Esther;
- Ross (son) and Michelle have two daughters—June and Evie.

Toby will tell you that his family brings him more joy than any one man could ever ask for. In his free time, he enjoys fishing, reading, spending time on the water, writing, and gardening.

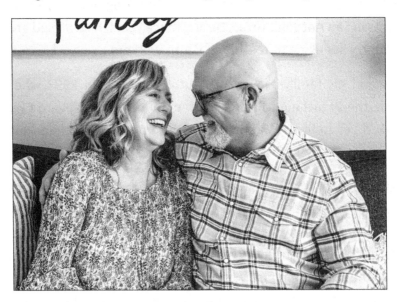

Toby continues to serve as the Lead Pastor for Cross Timbers and has authored several books including, *Living the Dream, The Great Adventure, God Drives Me Crazy, Normal, It Is Well*, and *Harvest*.

If you found this book helpful, we invite you to leave a review on Amazon. Your review will help others find this book and be able to experience this freedom-stirring message.

— Thank You

You can follow Toby on Twitter:

@tobyslough

Find him on Facebook:

www.facebook.com/tobyslough

Hear him speak:

www.crosstimberschurch.org

Invite him to speak:

www.NotYetTheBook.com

www.tobyslough.com

PEACE IS POSSIBLE,
JESUS IS REAL,
AND YOUR BEST DAYS
ARE YET AHEAD

Made in the USA
Coppell, TX
26 January 2020